# Gluten-free the Right Way!

## Gluten-free . Dairy-free . GMO-free

Avoid the Common Mistakes
of Eating Gluten-free so
You and Your Family Can Heal
and Feel Your Best

Sharon K. Harmon, PhD

**Gluten-free the Right Way!**
Avoid Common Mistakes of Eating Gluten-free so You Can Truly Heal and Feel Your Best

Published by Sharon Harmon, Life Design for Health, LLC

ISBN: 979-8-9919543-0-3 (paperback)
ISBN: 979-8-9919543-1-0 (ebook)

Edited by: Raven Petty

www.sharonharmon.com

The information provided in this book and on the website is designed to provide helpful information on the subjects discussed. It is for educational purposes only, not medical advice, and in no way should anyone infer that we are practicing medicine. This book is not meant to be used, nor should it be used, to diagnose or treat any medical condition. For diagnosis or treatment of any medical problem, consult your physician or other qualified healthcare professional. The publisher and author are not responsible for any specific health or allergy needs that may require medical supervision and are not liable for any damages or negative consequences from any treatment, action, application, or preparation, to any person reading or following the information in this book. We recommend that you do your own independent research before using or purchasing anything. References are provided for informational purposes only and do not constitute endorsement of any websites or other sources. Readers should be aware that the website links in this book may change.

# Dedication

This book is dedicated to my mom, Rita Koomen. I know you are looking down and smiling as you see my first of many health-related books come to fruition. It started with you!

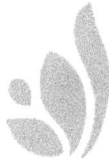

# Contents

# Acknowledgments

First and foremost, I want to thank my mom who first taught me that food is healing as it healed our family many years ago. It started me on my journey to holistic health.

Thanks as well to my husband and son, Chris and Zach, who allowed me to learn and experiment with them as we went through our personal gluten-free journey.
You taught me much as well.

I also want to thank my clients and students, too many to name, who continue to educate me as we work together. This, ironically, included my editor who read through my manuscript as a gluten-free newbie and provided some valuable feedback.
Thank you, Raven!

And, finally, thank you, dear reader. May your gluten-free journey be a more direct one, with the help of the information in this book!

# How to Use This Book

You may be sensitive to gluten and not realize it. This is not uncommon as gluten is difficult to digest for many people.

However, if you are eating it daily, you don't notice it because it is your current normal. You may always be tired or have some brain fog, for example, but don't equate that to the food you eat. It could show up as a variety of physical symptoms as well as mental and emotional symptoms, as explained in this book.

Many people benefit when they remove gluten from their diet. It could be a short-term healing strategy or a life-long lifestyle choice because it makes you feel better.

When you remove gluten, you are giving your body more energy to work on other things, allowing your body to heal and/or repair itself. After reading this book, you may discover there are other possible culprit foods you want to reduce or eliminate as well.

## Our Family Story

In the early 2000s, gluten was not on my radar. Not sure if anyone was talking about it back then. I knew I did better when eating less bread, as my skin would break out less often, but that was it.

If I think back to growing up, my mom also saw a grain connection. When we had oatmeal for breakfast, she always prepared herself millet cereal instead. She just felt better without the oatmeal, likely because, as you will learn, oatmeal has gluten in it.

My family's gluten story started when our son was almost two years old. He would have coughing episodes after eating certain foods. It was especially noticeable after eating out at a popular sandwich restaurant.

Not only did he have a coughing episode, but the next day he invariably had a temper tantrum, something that was extremely rare for him. We finally determined that it was the whole-grain baguette that caused the more severe reaction.

After doing more research and experimenting at home, I determined the culprit was the gluten in several different grains.

So, we started cutting gluten out of our son's diet. On the rare occasion, when he did have gluten, it was like clockwork. The day after, our son would have a meltdown. Invariably, he would have an episode of crying or a temper tantrum, which was not like him.

Gluten can do that – it can affect you shortly after a meal, the next day, and even a week after eating it. That is when we went totally gluten-free. At least he did.

Eventually, I started getting stricter myself.

Up to that point, I had been limiting my breads and grains. However, one thing I still ate was sprouted wheat bread because at that time, it was thought that a grain that had been sprouted greatly reduced the effects of the grain, including the gluten.

We now know that is not true. I weaned myself off the sprouted bread, but when I did eat a piece, I could tell my body did not like it. It affected my heart rate immediately – I could feel my heart beating faster. It also affected my brain, making it harder to concentrate, for up to 48 hours. And, it made me more tired the next day. So, I decided to completely remove gluten too. What a difference!

## What About You?

There are now tests available to see if you are gluten-sensitive, which I discuss in Chapter 2. However, another way to determine if gluten is a problem for you or your child is to eliminate all forms of gluten for 2 to 4 weeks (see Chapter 2), after which you eat a small amount of gluten on purpose and monitor your reaction.

Most people are very surprised that they get a reaction, which will vary for each person as explained in Chapter 1. However, what you need to know is there is a right way to go gluten-free and a wrong way.

When you remove gluten products, you want to substitute them with healthy alternatives. Many processed gluten-free products have suspect ingredients and are not very nutritious. You also want to consider rotating the gluten-free alternatives you use, so you do not create another health problem, like oxalate issues or nut sensitivities. More about this in Chapter 4.

The good news is there are many more gluten-free products available since the time my family went gluten-free. Chapter 5 will explain how to negotiate these many options, what to look for, and what to avoid when you shop.

And, if you like to bake, Chapter 6 will show you how to substitute your typical ingredients with gluten-free ones so you can continue to use some of your favorite recipes.

Use this book to get up-to-speed on why to go gluten-free, and then learn how to do it the right way, avoiding the learning curve I had when I got started. Once you get the basics down, you will realize it is easier than you think.

# Getting Started

I suggest **reading this book all the way through** before jumping into your gluten-free adventure. At least read Chapters 1 through 4, as you will get a better idea of what types of products can contain gluten—it can hide in many places and not just food.

I want you to avoid the mistakes I made as an early adopter of a gluten-free lifestyle.

Chapter 4 will provide additional tips so you do not fall into the typical trap of substituting gluten foods with others that may eventually cause different problems. Plus, I give you some tips when eating out at restaurants and family functions. And, you will find Chapters 5 and 6 very useful once you start shopping and baking gluten-free.

**Creating a support team around you** will be helpful as you work through the steps in this book and try new foods and recipes. Having a spouse or loved one, a friend, or a parent with similar-aged children who also wants to go gluten-free can be very beneficial. Support each other, shop and cook together, have a fermenting party, etc.

It is also a **good idea to keep a journal**. Record any health problems you hope to correct, whether they are physical, mental, or emotional. Keep records of when you started going gluten-free, GMO-free, dairy/casein-free, etc., and what health-related changes occur as you move forward. If you accidentally "get glutened," record those dates too so you can get a good idea of how gluten affects you.

There is much you can do on your own. However, if you find that health issues improve for a while and eventually level out,

**consider seeing a holistic healthcare practitioner**, especially one that understands the complexity of food and other lifestyle factors that may be hindering you (as explained in Chapter 2).

Certain supplements can also help accelerate the healing process. And, if you have been gluten-sensitive for a while, you may be deficient in some nutrients. The right practitioner can help you determine which nutrients are needed, as well as determine if specific toxins, infections, or other lifestyle issues need to be resolved for optimal health.

Use this book to get educated so you can **become your own health advocate or that for your child**. If you need to work with a practitioner, you want to be partners in your health journey as you are the best judge of your body and your child's body.

Summaries are provided at the end of each chapter to assist you.

# CHAPTER 1

# Why Eat Gluten-free?

Many celiac and gluten-literate doctors believe that gluten sensitivity is more widespread than we realize. Some, like Dr. Alessio Fasano, who is one of the leading gluten sensitivity researchers, believes that all humans have a problem digesting gluten. It just shows up differently in different people.

That might be true, but I believe there are other factors involved.

Part of it has to do with how gluten-containing grains such as wheat are grown, harvested, processed, etc. For example, in other countries where wheat is grown differently, gluten sensitivity is not as prevalent. I have met many Americans over the years who have traveled to Europe and eaten wheat products there without any of their normal reactions, myself included.

A person's overall health and other lifestyle choices must also be considered.

However, I have seen it many times, **removing gluten from your diet and lifestyle can be a game changer**, especially if you are not feeling well or you feel stuck in your healing journey.

This chapter will cover the many effects of gluten on the body and why you may want to eliminate gluten from your diet, even temporarily. Yes, it directly affects the gut, but the consequences of this gut reaction to the rest of the body can be quite extensive, emotionally and mentally as well.

Each person is different, so learning all the possible effects will help you negotiate your own reaction and how you want to move forward in your journey.

After looking at potential side effects, I will discuss gluten in more detail and why it can affect the body. There may be more reasons than just the gluten itself. You will also learn about its addictive qualities as well as other foods that may cause similar reactions. All things you need to know to go gluten-free the right way.

## Gluten-related Health Problems

Until more recently, gluten was mostly associated with **Celiac Disease**, an autoimmune disease, which directly affects the small intestine. A person with Celiac Disease has very specific symptoms that occur if they eat even a hint of gluten. They are not able to tolerate any gluten.

Now, many doctors agree that there are quite a few health issues that can occur because of gluten. This is called being **gluten sensitive**, where the reaction is often more delayed. It is also sometimes called non-celiac gluten sensitivity. (The term gluten intolerant is often usually used interchangeably to describe Celiac Disease and gluten sensitivity.)

In the past, it was thought that Celiac Disease was strictly genetic, but now it is believed that it can start as a gluten sensitivity that goes unchecked. Therefore, it is also a lifestyle-based disease, which is another good reason to determine if you are gluten-sensitive, as I will explain later in this book.

What is becoming more recognized is how gluten contributes to a variety of **autoimmune diseases**, not just Celiac Disease. This includes autoimmune thyroid diseases (Grave's and Hashimoto's), Rheumatoid Arthritis, Type 1 Diabetes, Irritable Bowel Syndrome (IBS), Chronic Fatigue, and Fibromyalgia, just to name a few. There are over 100 autoimmune diseases with more added every year!

Gluten sensitivity tends to **directly affect the gut lining**; however, symptoms can present in many different areas of the body. In fact, Dr. Steven Gundry, cardiothoracic surgeon and author of *Plant Paradox*, explains that all autoimmune patients he sees also have gut issues, including gluten antibodies, even if the patient is not complaining about their digestive system.

Gluten also **creates inflammation in the body** and can be a factor in many other health issues, some of which you might not expect.

For example, triple-board certified internist and hypertension specialist, Dr. Mark Houston in Nashville, TN, believes gluten sensitivity plays a factor in numerous cardiovascular illnesses. Dr. David Perlmutter, board-certified neurologist and author of *Grain Brain*, considers gluten a **brain irritant and a neurotoxin**.

Many potential symptoms are listed below.

If you have an autoimmune disease or recognize yourself or your child in some of the **gluten-related symptoms**, you may want to consider removing gluten from the diet, even for a few weeks (as explained in Chapter 2), to see if there is improvement.

- Gas and bloating
- Stomach or intestinal pain, including IBS

- Nausea and vomiting, especially projectile vomiting
- Acid-reflux, heartburn, or GERD (gluten can damage the acid-producing cells of the stomach)
- Constipation and/or diarrhea
- Anemia (iron, folic acid, or B-12 deficiency) causing weakness, fatigue, shortness of breath, pallor, lightheadedness, and a fast heartbeat
- Joint pain such as dull ache or sudden stabbing pain
- Muscle cramps
- Brain fog, concentration problems, and dementia
- Mood changes, such as anxiety or depression
- Headaches, migraines, and seizures
- Bone pain and bone loss, including osteopenia and osteoporosis
- Fatigue and weakness
- Unexplained bouts of dizziness, loss of balance (Ataxia), or ear-ringing
- Neuropathy (feeling of numbness or tingling), especially in hands and feet
- Heart palpitations
- Asthma-like symptoms
- Acne and skin rashes, including dermatitis herpetiformis, eczema, and psoriasis
- Hormone imbalance, including testosterone problems in men
- Unexplained infertility and miscarriage
- Unexplained weight loss or weight gain
- Dental enamel defects, cavities, and crooked teeth
- Painful tongue or mouth ulcers
- A child's failure to thrive or shortened stature
- Hyperactivity, Attention Deficit Disorder (ADD), Attention Deficit Hyperactivity Disorder (ADHD), and Autism
- Bipolar Disorder and Schizophrenia

Dr. Rodney Ford, a gluten-free pediatrician in New Zealand, started finding gluten sensitivities in children over 30 years ago, especially in children with allergies. Other common symptoms he correlates in **children who are gluten sensitive** include eczema and skin rashes, constipation and/or diarrhea, acid reflux, recurring tummy aches, vomiting, migraines and other headaches, and chronic hives. He also includes the sickly child who is often tired and grumpy.

Learning disorders and general "failure to thrive" issues may also be helped by removing gluten (and/or other culprit foods) from the diet.

Additionally, it is important to note that gluten **sensitivities often occur generationally**. If you are gluten sensitive it is likely that (1) one of your parents are/were gluten sensitive and/or (2) one or more of your children are (or will be) gluten sensitive. You can often look at your extended family and see similarities in illnesses and health issues, not unlike my family as I described in the Introduction.

## What is Gluten?

Before getting into the details of how gluten affects the body, let's look at where gluten can be found. It is not always clear. For example, gluten sensitivity typically refers to the effects of wheat gluten. But, did you know that all grains that form a seed contain some amount of gluten?

Some grains contain gluten that is more similar to wheat gluten and are typically eliminated in a gluten-free diet.

The **most common gluten-containing grains** that must be eliminated are wheat (including typical white bread), barley (including malt), rye, and other wheat-based grains such as spelt, durum, semolina, Kamut®, einkorn, and teff. (Some are considered "ancient" grains and might have less gluten but can still be a problem when trying to heal.) Couscous, bulgur, and brewer's yeast are included too.

Grains (or seeds) that are most **typically considered gluten-free include** rice, quinoa, millet, buckwheat, and amaranth. However, more sensitive people might also be sensitive to the lower gluten content in some of these and may need to consider going grain-free (as discussed in Chapter 3).

**Oats, corn, and soy are also usually considered gluten-free, but there are other concerns** to be considered. Oats and oat flour, for example, still contain gluten. It is different from wheat gluten, but if you are sensitive, like me, it can be a problem. (You can check yourself using an elimination diet, explained in Chapter 2.)

Oats are also often "cross-contaminated" because they are typically processed in the same facility as wheat. You can get oats that are labeled "gluten-free" (meaning they are processed in a separate facility and not tainted by wheat gluten), which would be the best option if you are not sensitive to oats.

Corn and soy, on the other hand, contain proteins that are very similar to gluten. The protein in soy, for instance, is digested by the same enzyme as wheat gluten. Corn contains a form of gluten as well. In addition, both corn and soy are typically genetically modified (GM) or GM-tainted. The Bt-toxin found in GM corn and the abundant pesticides found in GM foods in general can present very similar symptoms to wheat gluten when eaten.

To be truly healthy, GM foods (and related gene-edited foods) should be removed from everyone's diet, not only when converting to a gluten-free diet. This will be discussed in more detail in later chapters. (You can also learn more about GMOs at *www.responsibletechnology.org.*)

## How Gluten Affects Your Body

From the many symptoms listed earlier, you can see that gluten can cause much more than digestive problems.

Gluten, and the other culprit foods, can cause problems in various parts of the body, including the brain. It can affect your emotions and mental health. I would add spiritual reactions, as well, since a "foggy brain" can hinder your ability for deep prayer and/or meditation.

It is the proteins in the gluten that are the problem. Wheat gluten, for example, contains over 10 different proteins. Any of these proteins can essentially cause a problem, however, gliadin is the protein that most commonly creates health issues. Our bodies cannot fully digest gliadin. Instead, it responds by creating an **over-production of "zonulin"** in the gut.

Zonulin is a protein that helps to anchor the cells in the intestinal lining so they are held close together. However, when gluten is eaten and zonulin production becomes elevated, it causes the cells to spread apart, creating what is called **intestinal permeability or "leaky gut."**

This, in turn, allows food-based proteins (or food particles) to travel through the gut wall into the bloodstream, where they are not supposed to be. The immune system sees these proteins as enemies and attempts to fight them off.

If this occurs in a healthy person, the immune cells can attack these foreign bodies and be done with it.

However, continually eating gluten does not give your body a break. Or, if your health is compromised and your immune system is already overworked, the **immune cells can start attacking** other parts of the body too.

This will also occur if you are eating so many gluten-containing foods (including culprit foods like corn, soy, and GMOs) that it becomes too much for your body to handle. Other health issues start to surface.

In some cases (such as Celiac Disease), collateral damage occurs in the **small intestine where "villous atrophy" occurs**. The villi are small hair-like tentacles that line the intestinal wall and help absorb nutrients during digestion. When these become damaged, malabsorption of nutrients occurs, resulting in deficiencies of vitamins, minerals, etc.

(I believe this can occur in gluten-sensitive people as well, which is why gluten sensitivity can eventually result in Celiac Disease in some people. There may be a connection to recurring Small Intestinal Bacterial Overgrowth (SIBO) as well.)

When the immune cells start attacking other parts of the body, it can cause inflammation and ultimately lead to an autoimmune disease. **The resulting symptoms and where they occur in the body will depend on the person and their inherent weaknesses.** For example, the resulting inflammation may occur in the joints, causing joint pain, the nerves, causing nerve damage, and the skin, causing skin issues.

Zonulin also controls the **blood-brain barrier permeability**. That is why gluten sensitivity can cause brain-related symptoms such as "brain fog" and dementia. Some experts believe that gluten directly affects the nerves in the gut more than the intestinal lining, causing gluten-induced neuropathy such as ataxia, vertigo, and tremors, as well as a diagnosis of Bi-polar Disorder or Schizophrenia.

## Addictive Effects of Gluten (and Dairy)

Digestion problems and inflammation inside the body, resulting from gluten sensitivity, do not always show up as obvious health issues right away. It can be especially difficult to figure out in young children who cannot verbalize how they feel. However, if a gluten sensitivity is not addressed at a younger age, it can potentially result in more health problems later in life.

One common sign that a young child is gluten-sensitive is their selection of foods. Do you know someone who only eats grains (like bread and pasta) and dairy (like cheese and milk) and refuses most other foods? Do their typical meals consist primarily of "white" foods?

In a gluten-sensitive person, these foods are not properly broken-down during digestion and actually **create opiate-type compounds** in the body. These compounds mimic the effects of morphine, which can dramatically affect the nervous system and the brain, as well as other parts of the body. (MSG and other food preservatives can do this as well.)

This reaction results in strong cravings to grains and dairy, so that a young gluten-sensitive child typically does not want to have other foods when offered. They are literally feeding their addiction.

Common symptoms in these types of children include: high pain tolerance, inattention and/or spacey behavior, aggression, stimming, mood changes, poor eye contact, difficulty speaking, as well as anxiety, depression, and irritability.

This cycle can be broken.

Ultimately, when you substitute the "normal" foods with gluten-free (or grain-free) and dairy-free options, thereby reducing the opiate-like reaction, children will often open up to other food options and start eating more vegetables, animal products, etc. However, the process is not always straightforward, and you may need the support of a gluten-literate practitioner as well as your spouse and other friends or family members.

It can sometimes be confusing for you and your child as you negotiate the process of going gluten-free. (See more in Introduction.)

Just like any other addiction, there can be a withdrawal period that makes you or your child very uncomfortable, physically, mentally, and/or emotionally. You may need to make adjustments as you move forward and possibly address nutrient deficiencies.

Zinc deficiency, for example, can be a sign of picky eating. Other common deficiencies that can result from both picky eating and gluten sensitivity include folate, iron, magnesium, niacin, riboflavin, and thiamin as well as certain vitamins. A good practitioner can help you figure this out.

Next, we will explore why gluten sensitivity is on the rise and how to determine if you are gluten-sensitive. Chapter 2 will also discuss additional ways to heal the gut long-term.

## Chapter 1 Summary

∞ Gluten sensitivity is different from a severe allergy or Celiac Disease. A sensitivity can create a more delayed reaction and often creates symptoms that are physical as well as emotional and mental. (See detailed list in Chapter 1.)

∞ Gluten sensitivities can lead to autoimmune symptoms and possibly even Celiac Disease. Some symptoms may be more specific to children and can often occur generationally.

∞ The most common gluten-containing grains that should be eliminated from a gluten-free diet include wheat and other wheat-based grains such as spelt, durum, semolina, Kamut®, einkorn, and teff as well as barley (including malt), rye, couscous, bulgur, and brewer's yeast. Oats need to be eliminated too.

∞ Grain and seed flours most commonly considered gluten-free (or very low in gluten) include rice, quinoa, millet, buckwheat, and amaranth. (See Chapter 6 for grain-free flour options.)

∞ All forms of corn and soy should also be eliminated in a gluten-free diet as they contain similar proteins; plus they are commonly genetically modified (GMO crops).

∞ When eaten, gluten affects the body by creating an overproduction of "Zonulin" in the gut, which can lead to intestinal permeability (or leaky gut), compromised immune system, small intestine issues, and blood-brain barrier permeability.

∞ Gluten and dairy can be addictive due to the opiate-like compounds created by the body when digestion is compromised; a key reason why dairy should be eliminated (even temporarily) during a gluten-free diet.

CHAPTER 2

# Determining Your Sensitivity

As mentioned previously, gluten sensitivities are more prevalent in some countries than others. And, as you have probably already figured out, **each person reacts differently to gluten, some worse than others**. That is because each of us is different.

Your health history, your generational weaknesses, and your lifestyle choices make your body unique. These factors can also contribute to your sensitivities, as we will explore in this chapter.

We will also look at different ways you can determine if you are gluten-sensitive. We will review some testing options as well as introduce the concept of a 2- to 4-week gluten elimination trial. For some people, that is all they need, especially if their symptoms are milder, to determine the best direction going forward.

The end of the chapter will explore the concept of healing gluten sensitivity, looking at the digestive system and other factors.

Ultimately, you want to figure out how many of your health problems are connected to gluten, or possibly one of the other food culprits discussed. The goal is to heal the body.

**The body is made to repair itself**, but often we get in our own way.

The more information you have, the better decisions you can make moving forward, so that you can go gluten-free the right way.

## The Rise in Gluten Sensitivity

People have become more sensitive to gluten in recent years. There are several reasons for this increase.

First, the gluten we eat today is **not the same gluten our grandparents ate**. In the United States, for example, wheat has been "selectively bred" over the years for specific traits such as taste, texture, rise, high-yielding, and drought tolerance. (It is the gluten that gives bread its fluffy, chewy, and stretchy qualities.)

This breeding has caused the gluten in wheat to become much more prevalent than wheat available 50 to 100 years ago.

Then there are the **additional chemicals**. It has been common for years to use pesticides on wheat and other grains during the growing process. However, for the past 25 years or so, especially in the United States, the toxic herbicide glyphosate (among others) is purposely used 7 to 10 days before harvesting to obtain a higher yield, drying up the crop for easier harvesting.

That means there is a high concentration of chemicals directly on the mature wheat kernels that are harvested. (See also GM Foods below.) Plus post-harvest, fungicides, and insecticides are often used to keep the grain free of mold and insects until it is time for processing.

All of these directly applied chemicals end up accumulating in your body, especially affecting the digestive system, when you eat the wheat.

However, it is not only the wheat that has changed. **Our bodies and our environment have changed** as well. Have you noticed that with each generation, the children seem to be more sensitive and less resilient?

Adults are feeling the effects too, as more illnesses and autoimmune diseases are occurring. Food quality, water quality, and air quality have all diminished over the years resulting in more toxins and stress in our environment.

The environment and the **lifestyle choices we make** can make a big impact on our overall health. Many of them greatly affect how sensitive we are to food, including gluten. Some even mimic gluten-like symptoms, especially pesticides and electromagnetic frequencies (EMFs), as you will see below.

*Poor Nutrition* – The foods we eat daily have a dramatic effect on the health of the cells, glands, and organs in our body. Quality foods and beverages equal a healthier body.

Processed foods are just not as nutritious as fresh, homemade foods. If we continually give it bad food and few nutrients, the digestive system will also suffer. Our stomach acid gets out of balance, our pancreas makes fewer digestive enzymes, and our intestines have fewer good bacteria.

The good news is that the body continuously regenerates itself. The more nutrients we can give the body, the better.

*Low-quality Water* – The water that comes out of the faucet in our homes is loaded with chemicals, microorganisms, fluoride, heavy metals, pesticides, etc., many of which compromise our immune and digestive systems. It may be a little better out of the refrigerator filter, but it has been proven that the filter housings often accumulate bacteria over time.

Most bottled water is not good either, especially since the plastic of the bottle can leach into the water. Instead, we should be drinking quality water either from a trusted natural spring or from a quality water filtration system. (For more information, see *www.sharonharmon.com/blog/quality-water*.)

**Genetically Modified (GM) Foods and Pesticides** – GM foods (or GMOs) were first introduced into the mainstream in the 1990s. The seeds for these foods are either engineered to withstand high amounts of pesticides and/or have been injected with the Bt-toxin, which is made to kill the bug if it tries to eat the plant.

This allows many more toxic pesticides to be sprayed on the crops, especially the herbicide called glyphosate.

Imagine the harm these toxins are creating in our bodies when we continuously eat the same plant. At a minimum, they compromise our good bacteria and gut flora, which in turn affects the digestive and immune systems. It also depletes certain nutrients in our body, such as minerals. More will be explained in Chapter 3. (Additional information about GMOs can also be found at *www.responsibletechnology.org*.)

**Pollution and Air Quality** – New chemicals are introduced into the environment daily. It is said that the average person has over 170 different toxins in their body at one given time. Our bodies are working so hard to eliminate the toxins we eat, breathe, smell, and touch (and put on our skin), that there is less energy for other body functions, such as digestion.

Pesticides are a large part of this, but so are products used on our body, in and around our home, in our cars, etc.

As you remove toxic products and exposures in your daily life, your body starts naturally eliminating some of them. Other toxins may get stored in certain parts of your body and need help to eliminate. (Check out *www.whatsonmyfood.org* for more information.)

***Electromagnetic Frequencies (EMFs)*** – Our exposure to EMFs and wireless radiation has dramatically increased since the 1990s, especially with the introduction of cell phones, cell towers and wireless (Wi-Fi) networks, Bluetooth devices, smart wearables, computerized cars, etc.

All of these devices affect how cells in our bodies absorb nutrients and eliminate toxins, causing many of the same symptoms as gluten in our bodies.

Even worse is using and wearing these devices so close to our stomach area, where our food gets digested. More recently, wireless radiation has been shown to act like an antibiotic in the body, so it can also affect the gut similar to GMOs and pesticides. (You can find more information in my *EMF Basics* article at *www.sharonharmon.com/blog/EMF-basics.*)

***Antibiotics*** – The overuse of antibiotics is another problem because they kill off the "good" bacteria at the same time it is going after the harmful bacteria. Even one round of antibiotics creates an imbalance in the gut microbiome, as well as other parts of the body.

We need good bacteria to help with digestion and absorption of nutrients. Rebuilding the gut after the use of antibiotics can take a while. It is important as the correct balance is the key to optimal immune system health.

***Other Pharmaceuticals*** – Other medications can also compromise our digestive system and gut flora. At a minimum, this includes contraceptives, acne medicines (like Accutane and Tetracycline), steroids, nonsteroidal anti-inflammatory drugs (NSAIDs) used to reduce pain (like aspirin, ibuprofen, naproxen), proton-pump inhibitors, as well as your basic acid-blocking medications and vaccines.

***Microbes and Infections*** – Undetected low-grade infections from microbes, such as bacteria, viruses, parasites, and fungi, also weaken the immune system. Things like Lyme-related illnesses and mold exposure are two common culprits. An undetected dental infection is another.

Microbes can also get stuck in the digestive tract, including the gut lining, and cause digestive havoc. (Sometimes this happens after taking an antibiotic.) It can become a no-win situation unless these microbes and/or infections are also addressed.

***Stress, Trauma, and Strenuous Exercise*** – It is normal to experience stress once in a while, but if there is a big stressor, like a death in the family or losing a job, it can take a toll on your body in many ways. Unresolved traumas and emotional triggers can too.

It is also shown that continuous strenuous exercise, including endurance sports, can cause intestinal damage. Your body does not perform optimally when under constant stress, which in turn compromises many systems in your body, including your digestive system.

If your body is inundated by any of the environmental and/or lifestyle factors listed above, your digestive system becomes compromised, making it harder to digest gluten (and other foods) and absorb the nutrients it needs.

**The more you can clean up and/or modify these other areas of your life, the stronger your body will be.** Granted, some of these toxic lifestyle habits are easier to shift than others. However, the more toxins, potential infections, and stress you can reduce, the better chance you have to heal your gut and eventually reintroduce gluten or other culprit food.

If you have multiple lifestyle changes you need to make, you may need the support of a holistic health practitioner and/or lifestyle coach to help you prioritize.

## Testing for Gluten Sensitivity

You read in Chapter 1 the many symptoms gluten can create in the body when there is a gluten sensitivity. There are many levels of sensitivity, with the extreme being gluten intolerance in Celiac Disease.

On the other hand, if you are gluten-sensitive, your symptoms will be unique to you. (If you suspect you have Celiac Disease, be sure to consult a celiac-literate practitioner as a biopsy of the small intestine is usually required for confirmation.)

Until more recently, gluten sensitivity was difficult to diagnose. **Previous medical testing was not that accurate**, often resulting in false negatives because the blood test concentrated on just one component of the gluten, the gliadin, and measured for the resulting gliadin antibody (antigliadin).

This test (and others like biopsies and DNA testing) can often detect the gluten intolerance found in Celiac Disease, but not necessarily the more common gluten sensitivities. Stool tests can also be limiting, as they only check for gliadin antibodies in the intestine, rather than throughout the whole body.

As explained in the previous chapter, there are multiple components (proteins and peptides) of wheat, and these should all be checked. **More comprehensive blood (and saliva) tests** were first developed by Cyrex Labs, which is still one of the premier gluten-testing labs.

When a Cyrex "Array 3" lab test is done, for example, over 10 peptides of wheat (not just gliadin) are analyzed, so you get a good picture of your grain sensitivities. The "Array 2" panel will pinpoint if you already have intestinal permeability (leaky gut).

The Cyrex "Array 4" panel checks for gluten-associated cross-reactive foods and food sensitivities, which may be helpful for those who find themselves sensitive to many types of foods. (To see all the available tests, go to *www.cyrexlabs.com*. See also Resources in the back of this book for additional testing options.)

**Genetic testing (also called DNA testing)** is another available option that can determine if a person carries specific genes linked to a higher likelihood of developing a gluten sensitivity. This can be helpful information. However, I am not a big fan of genetic testing as people often get fixated on their results. Having a specific gene does not dictate an illness; your lifestyle does.

As Dr. Bruce Lipton explains in his book, *The Biology of Belief*, when we create a healthy environment around us, we will not activate the genes that create disease. Even more importantly, we can inactivate the genes that are causing us problems and return to health.

The big take-a-way is that **you don't necessarily need a lab test** to determine if you are gluten-sensitive. Instead, you can do a 2- to 4-week gluten elimination trial as explained next.

# Gluten Elimination Trial

One of the best ways to determine if you have a gluten sensitivity, without a lab test, is to **temporarily remove gluten from your diet and then reintroduce it,** as you monitor your reactions. This is commonly called a "2-week gluten elimination diet," but it usually takes a minimum of 3 to 4 weeks to complete.

For some of you, it may be the first time you truly pay attention to how your body reacts to different foods. It can be an eye-opening experience!

During the elimination period, you completely remove gluten from your diet for 2 weeks. You may also decide to eliminate 1 or more of the other gluten-like culprits that I talk about in this book. At the end of the 2 weeks, you slowly reintroduce the gluten-based foods while monitoring your reactions.

**The goal is to monitor your reactions before, during, and after the elimination** to get a good picture of what is happening in the body.

If you have many health problems and digestive issues, it may be best to work with a gluten-literate practitioner who knows how to conduct elimination diets. Eliminating too many foods at once may be too much for your body.

On the other hand, if you are doing this more out of curiosity, you may want to restrict more of the gluten-based foods and/or cross-reactive foods, so you can get a really good idea of the main culprits as you slowly reintroduce.

The most common gluten-related culprit foods would include gluten (and oats), dairy, corn, and soy.

Keep in mind that the more foods you eliminate, the longer it will take to do the reintroduction period. This may be too restrictive for your current state of health without adding supplements. Alternatively, you can do a separate elimination trial for each suggested food. Nevertheless, it would be best to at least eliminate gluten and dairy in an initial elimination, since they create very similar reactions in the body, which can be especially noticeable in children.

Below is a summary of the process, broken down into three main steps.

**STEP 1: Before Getting Started** – Preparation is key. Use this book to **understand what "gluten-free" entails**. Get familiar with gluten-based grains versus "gluten-free" options, which foods can be cross-reactive, and which processed foods tend to have hidden gluten (as explained in Chapter 3). You may also need to temporarily remove certain body products, supplements, and other products in the house (see Chapter 4).

Take your time and **make sure you have everything you need in the house** before beginning the elimination. You can also use the many meal and snack suggestions in Chapter 3.

Optimally, it would be best to not travel or eat out during this time, so you are not tempted by your favorite foods. Cross-contamination can easily happen when food preparation is out of your control. If you eat gluten-related food by accident, it is best to start over.

It is also best to **write down all your health-related symptoms** before you get started. Think of anything physically going on, as well as emotional and mental issues using the information in Chapter 1.

Believe it or not, it can be difficult to remember how you felt even after 2 weeks, especially if many of your symptoms go away. Once you have your symptom list, stop all gluten-related foods and products.

*STEP 2: During the Elimination Period* – Eliminate all culprit foods. At least **eliminate all gluten-containing foods** (including hidden gluten) if you are just checking for gluten sensitivities. If you are checking for reactions to dairy (or any other cross-reactive food), remove that type of food from your diet as well.

In these 2 weeks, you will not eliminate the gliadin antibodies, as explained in Chapter 1, but **you should see a reduction of symptoms**. There is the possibility that you feel worse for the first couple of days before you start feeling better, as your body eliminates and adjusts itself.

Pay attention to the changes in your body.

At the 2-week mark, before reintroducing any gluten (or other culprit food), review **your initial list of symptoms** and see what changed. Have you had more energy? How is your brain fog? Are you sleeping better? Have you been less emotional or moody? Are your bowel movements different?

*STEP 3: Start Reintroduction* – The reintroduction part is just as important as taking the 2-week break from gluten. **Reintroduce some gluten in the morning on day 15**, preferably on a day that you will be home, so you can monitor yourself closely.

Maybe eat a small portion of your favorite wheat bread for breakfast. Eat it just once and see what happens during the day. (The rest of your food should continue to be gluten-free.) Do this for 3 days, slightly increasing the portion each morning. You do not want to inundate your body but rather **monitor your reaction**.

Remember, it is not uncommon for food-related reactions to take place 1 to 3 days after eating the food (even up to 8 days!), especially when you consider things like sleep reactions, mental clarity, bowel movements, and mood. Write down (1) the food you ate and when you ate it, and (2) your reaction(s) and when they occurred. This will give you a good before and after "picture" that you can use to decide how you want to move forward.

After 3 days, stop the gluten-based test food and **continue to monitor your reactions, while you go back to eating gluten-free** (and free of other culprit foods) for the rest of the week. Then, if you also eliminated dairy, do the same thing on day 22: Reintroduce a dairy product, like milk or cheese, each morning for 3 days, monitoring your reaction. Then stop again for the rest of the week.

By the end of week 4, you should have a good indication of how you reacted to the main foods you eliminated.

For some, gluten sensitivity will be very obvious. For many, additionally eliminating dairy for the 2 weeks will help even more as gluten and dairy both cause similar brain, nervous system, and gut reactions in the body (see Chapter 1).

If you want to take it a step further, remove GM crops like corn and soy, as these foods also cause a high number of food reactions as well. (Note that, especially for children, other common food allergens include eggs, tree nuts, peanuts, sesame, and shellfish.)

**The ultimate goal is to find your culprit food(s), not just gluten, so that long-term you only need to eliminate a minimal number of foods,** since eliminating too many healthy foods can potentially result in nutrient deficiencies.

Consider working with a good holistic health practitioner to make sure you get a balanced diet that is right for your body. This may be especially helpful if you are having challenging health issues.

No two people are the same, so consider your particular situation. (A good resource that can provide more detail is *The Elimination Diet* by Alissa Segersten and Tom Malterre.)

NOTE: *I am also a big advocate of muscle testing to help you determine the optimal foods for yourself and/or your family. Some practitioners know how to do this. If you want to learn how to muscle test yourself, go to www.sharonharmon.com/courses for my online course* Muscle Test with Confidence.

## Healing the Gut Long-term

If you find that gluten is a huge trigger food for you, you will want to eliminate it for a longer period. This is especially important to heal the gut. The goal is to be 100% off gluten (including hidden sources) for the body to stop making the gliadin antibodies.

If you stop eating gluten but then have just a little of it one day, the antibodies are reintroduced, and you essentially need to start all over again. (More about hidden sources and cross-contamination in Chapters 3 and 4.) You may not feel an immediate reaction, but the body is likely still affected.

**Eliminating gluten and GMOs (including corn and soy) is a great first step** and many people feel dramatically better after eliminating these. Some find that certain symptoms they have been living with for years dissipate after only a few weeks. (Dairy may need to be eliminated too, as explained in Chapter 1.)

In reality, **most people need to stay off gluten for 6 to 18 months** and sometimes other culprit foods, depending on the situation.

It is not enough for only the symptoms to go away temporarily. The **goal is to heal the intestinal lining and the blood-brain barrier** – to heal the inflammation that is occurring inside the body for a more permanent solution.

Quicker improvements are sometimes seen in people with more intestinal-related health issues like IBS, Crohn's, chronic constipation or diarrhea. Migraine headaches is another that can quickly resolve. For those with more chronic autoimmune conditions, it usually takes longer to improve and/or more fully heal.

For some people, staying off gluten and other key foods is all they need to do. For others, **additional steps may be necessary** to regain optimal health, especially when more complicated autoimmune factors are occurring.

These steps may include one or more of the following. Each person will be different based on their health history and lifestyle choices.

- Removing additional cross-reactive foods as explained in Chapter 4
- Replenishing depleted nutrients with specific supplements
- Eliminating infections caused by "cross-reactive" viruses, bacteria, fungi and/or parasites
- Identifying and removing specific environmental toxins (pesticides, plastics, chemicals, heavy metals, mold, mycotoxins, medications, etc.)
- Doing additional cleansing of the body
- Opening the channels of elimination (colon, liver, kidney, lungs, skin, lymph) for better detoxification

- Taking specific supplements to more fully heal the gut
- Clearing emotional blocks and past traumas
- Removing or replacing life stressors like a toxic job, over-exercise, hectic schedule, toxic relationships, etc.

Working with a holistic health practitioner who is gut-literate and gluten-literate can make a huge difference, especially if there is a complicated health history that may span more than a generation. A lifestyle coach can also help you make some adjustments.

In a perfect world, the goal would be to eat gluten (and/or dairy) again. This may not be realistic for everyone, but most people can reintroduce certain foods.

For example, after I got to a certain point (after a few years), I was able to eat organic einkorn sourdough bread once in a while without an issue. Einkorn is an ancient wheat that has not been modified like more traditional wheat grains, so it can be better tolerated by some.

However, overall, I continue to remain gluten-free (and mostly dairy-free) as I feel better when I do. I have more energy too.

I know other people who can eat their own baked goods using quality wheat flour from other countries, like Italy, where GMOs and pesticides are not as prevalent; or, eat homemade bread using organic wheat berries they grind themselves.

As a teenager, our son started eating all sorts of gluten-filled foods with little to no observable effect, but we had spent years off of gluten and dairy with gut-healing supplements to get to that point. However, he knows this is a "weak link" in his body and what his reactions are. If he starts feeling similar symptoms again, he knows where to start his healing journey.

In the next chapter, we will delve into the details of going gluten-free. The first step is to prepare yourself mentally and come up with a game plan so the actual process goes smoothly. This will be explained in Chapter 3.

# Chapter 2 Summary

∞ There are many reasons for the rise in gluten sensitivity, starting with years of selective breeding and genetic modification of the wheat seed, as well as the increased use of pesticides and herbicides.

∞ Less than optimal lifestyle choices also affect how we digest gluten and/or react to it.

∞ These lifestyle choices include your overall food quality, the water you drink, the air you breathe, the medicines and supplements you take, your EMF and wireless device exposures, your toxin and/or infection thresholds, your trauma and stress levels, etc.

∞ Testing for gluten sensitivity can be confusing as there are many options. At a minimum, you want to test for multiple gluten-based proteins (not just gliadin). Other options include checking the intestinal permeability and additional food sensitivities. There is genetic testing as well.

∞ A gluten elimination trial can also be used to check gluten sensitivity. You eliminate gluten (and other culprit foods) for 2 weeks and slowly reintroduce one food at a time over 3 days, as you monitor your reactions. (See more explanation in Chapter 2.)

∞ Before removing gluten from your diet, it is best to be prepared. Read this book ahead of time, purchase the foods and ingredients you need, plan your meals, and write down all your health-related symptoms before you begin.

∞ During the 2-week elimination period, write down the foods you eliminated and track your symptoms. See what changes.

∞ When reintroducing foods, take it slow. Introduce one food at a time as you monitor your body's reaction physically as well as emotionally, mentally, and energetically.

∞ If you find you are gluten-sensitive (or sensitive to another culprit food), removing the food from the diet 6 to 18 months is key to repairing the digestive system. Working on lifestyle factors and other specific health challenges at the same time will greatly improve the results. (See list in Chapter 2.)

## CHAPTER 3

# How to Eat Gluten-free

Most people generally feel better when they remove gluten from their diet, whether they have a specific health issue or not, especially in the United States.

If you are dealing with specific health symptoms, eating gluten-free can often accelerate the healing process. Removing gluten especially helps with digestive issues, allergies, brain-related issues, and autoimmune diseases, but as you learned in Chapter 1, there are many other benefits.

However, **there is a right way to go gluten-free and a wrong way**.

I want to set you up for success. It is more than just removing wheat products. It is also more than buying a product that says "gluten-free," as not all of them are created equal.

You need additional information so you can avoid the common mistakes, as **many foods mimic the effects of gluten**. And, gluten can hide in unexpected places.

In this chapter, you will learn which additional foods and ingredients to avoid and the **many places gluten can hide in food**.

The last section will give you a **wide variety of meal and snack ideas** so you are better equipped for both the 2-week challenge and should you decide to eliminate gluten long-term. (Chapter 4 will discuss cross-reactive foods and other hidden sources of gluten, so read that as well before getting started.)

Once you are prepared, it is optimal to do the gluten elimination trial as explained in Chapter 2. If you do the challenge correctly, eliminating certain culprit foods in addition to gluten itself, not only will you know for sure if gluten is the issue, but it will prepare you for moving forward.

The gluten challenge gives you a taste of what a gluten-free lifestyle will be like, so you are more prepared to get started.

## What to Consider First

Going gluten-free does not need to be difficult. Admittedly, it can seem overwhelming at first, especially as you learn the concepts in this book. But, if you take a few steps at a time, you will be there before you know it.

Before eliminating all the gluten (and related foods and products), it is **optimal to have alternates in hand**. Many alternatives will be explained in this chapter and Chapter 4.

And remember, just because a product says "gluten-free," does not mean it is good for you.

To make up for the lack of gluten, which usually provides the fluffiness and texture in baked goods, additives are often used, including genetically modified (GM) ones (or GMOs) and other cross-reactive ingredients. More sweeteners are often added as well.

As you remove gluten from your diet, you want to make sure you are **replacing it with good nutritious options**, not more processed foods.

If you already cook primarily from scratch, it is a matter of **knowing what to substitute** for ingredients that you are already using. Below are a few examples. More ideas and meal suggestions are described later in this chapter. (How to shop and bake gluten-free will be explained in later chapters.)

- Replace standard or whole wheat pasta with brown rice pasta.
- Replace white flour or whole wheat flour with rice flour, garbanzo bean flour, and/or quinoa flour.
- Replace breadcrumbs in recipes with almond meal (in limited amounts) or ground flax seed.
- Replace breakfast cereals with prepared eggs or smoothies.
- Replace processed snack foods with vegetables and fruits and other more nutritious gluten-free snacks listed later in the chapter.

You also need to **consider your kitchen**. Gluten residue can be left behind on your countertops, cutting boards, ovens, toaster oven, etc.

It is best to do a full wipe down of everything in the kitchen and other eating surfaces before you get started. If you live by yourself, it will be easy to keep these surfaces gluten-free. It is more of a challenge in families where everyone is not eating gluten-free.

If the whole family eats gluten-free (at least at home), there will be **no cross-contamination** between gluten and gluten-free foods. You don't have to worry about gluten products contaminating things like butter or condiments, and there will be less preparation time overall.

The alternative is to consider having separate cutting boards and separate prep areas in the kitchen.

You may also want to consider a dedicated combination air-fryer/toaster oven, which can be used to heat a variety of foods. Over time, you will determine which gluten-free foods are acceptable to the whole family, limiting the number of gluten foods you need to prepare.

To truly benefit from eating gluten-free, it is optimal to be 100% committed.

If you remember from Chapter 1, eating gluten just once will cause your body to make the antigliadin (or other protein) antibodies again, and it can take a minimum of 3 to 6 months to get rid of them once more.

Slip-ups will happen and that is okay. Just keep in mind that the stricter you can be for a consistent period of time, the greater chance your gut has to heal.

Before we go any further, let's review the gluten-containing grains and the grains or seeds most often used as a substitute.

***Gluten-containing Grains to Eliminate*** – Grains that contain wheat-like gluten include wheat and wheat bran, barley and barley malt, rye, spelt, durum, semolina, Kamut®, einkorn, teff, durum, brewer's yeast, bulgur, couscous, as well as most commercial oats (as explained more in the next section).

***Grains (or Seeds) Considered Safe*** – When eating gluten-free the most common substitute grains (or seeds) include rice, quinoa, millet, buckwheat, and amaranth. Corn and soy are often included in this group as well; however, I would avoid them as explained in the next section.

## Cross-reactive Foods

"Cross-reactive" foods **have compounds that tend to mimic gluten**, which means it creates a similar reaction in the body as gluten, especially in the digestive system (or gut).

When eliminating gluten, it is important to at least eliminate soy and dairy/casein (due to similar protein digestion), oats, and GM foods like corn. The characteristics of these foods tend to make them the most cross-reactive, as explained below.

The cross-reactive food list below and the additional foods with hidden gluten listed in the next section are purposely comprehensive.

You need to know all the potential culprit foods, so you can see the many ways your food may be hurting you. These lists may also help explain why your current gluten-free lifestyle is not working optimally.

Don't worry or feel overwhelmed. Later in this chapter, I will give you many gluten-free, dairy-free, and GMO-free food and meal suggestions.

***Oats*** – Oats contain gluten. It is not the same as wheat gluten, but it is close enough that most people see better results when they also eliminate oats. That includes oat milk, oat yogurt, and other oat-based products, which should be avoided too, especially since these often contain questionable additives.

Oats are also one of the crops that is sprayed with the herbicide glyphosate prior to harvesting, which is additionally damaging to the gut (as explained in the last chapter). When you see packages of plain oatmeal that are labeled "gluten-free," this typically means that they have been processed in a facility that does not process wheat products, as the oats can also get cross-contaminated with wheat gluten. It does not necessarily mean they were grown and harvested without chemicals.

**Soy** – The protein in soy is broken down in the digestive system by the same enzyme as gluten, so it is often best to eliminate soy when going gluten-free. It gives your body a break.

Soy is also a genetically modified (GM) crop and, therefore, a high-pesticide crop found in many processed products like tofu, tempeh, soy milk, baked goods, etc. Some prepared soy products also contain wheat derivatives as will be explained in the next section.

***Genetically Modified (GM) Crops*** – One of the main herbicides, glyphosate, used on GM crops can mimic gluten sensitivity when eaten, so all GM foods should be removed from the diet as well.

GM corn and cotton, additionally contain the Bt-toxin, which makes them even more toxic to your body. (See Chapter 3 and 5 for more information on GMO foods.) **Corn contains a form of gluten as well**, so read your labels as ground corn is a common substitute for wheat in gluten-free products.

Processed gluten-free foods may contain flour from GM corn or soy as well as oils made from GM corn, soy, canola, and/or cottonseed oils. If a product contains one of these products or one of the other GM crops, such as sugar beets, alfalfa, or certain papaya, zucchini, and squash, be cautious.

At a minimum, make sure the packaged product includes a "NON-GMO Project" verified label. (You can find a list of non-GMO verified products at *www.nongmoproject.org*.) Using organic is the next best, although products can get tainted in the fields and during production. Eliminating GM crops is optimal, especially corn as it can often irritate the digestive system.

**Dairy (from Cow's Milk)** – Casein, one of the proteins in cow's milk, is broken down during digestion by the same enzyme as gluten. And like gluten, produces an opioid-type compound that can affect the nervous system, as explained in Chapter 1.

Additionally, most conventionally raised cows are fed GM grains. They too can get a "leaky gut," which means that gluten particles can get in their milk and ultimately into dairy products such as milk, cheese, and yogurt.

So, if your digestive system is already compromised, it would be beneficial to eliminate dairy too. Some sensitive people do okay with raw dairy because it still includes the enzymes necessary to digest the casein. Others can tolerate goat's milk. However, it is usually optimal to eliminate all dairy in the early stages.

How many of the above **foods you decide to eliminate** will depend on the status of your health and how far you want to take the healing process.

It also depends on which of these foods you currently eat most often, as it could potentially be your biggest culprit food other than gluten. This includes other grains typically considered gluten-free, like millet and rice, which can be considered "cross-reactive" in certain people.

What happens is that the body has become so busy attacking the gluten protein that it does not differentiate and starts attacking other proteins as well.

The body gets confused and starts making gluten antibodies for proteins other than wheat gluten.

This is less likely to occur if you work to eliminate the main cross-reactive foods listed above and you continue to **rotate the foods you keep in your diet**.

However, if you are not seeing the results for which you had hoped, you may want to consider removing all grains for a limited time. More grain-free products continue to become available, and there are many recipes now online using coconut flour, nuts and seeds, etc.

For especially sensitive people, there are still more foods that can be considered "cross-reactive." These cross-reactive foods include dried beans, seeds and seed flours, coffee and coffee beans, and other legumes like peanuts. The saponins and lectins in quinoa, for example, can irritate an already compromised digestive system.

For those who have multiple health problems and/or food allergies, it may require you to remove some of these other cross-reactive foods from your diets temporarily to give your digestive system a break.

It is **important not to eliminate too many foods for too long** as it can potentially create a nutrient deficiency.

Therefore, when it gets complicated, it is optimal to work with a holistic health practitioner to guide you, one who understands elimination diets and food sensitivities. The practitioner can also review your health history and lifestyle to see what other factors may be contributing to your gluten sensitivity (see Chapter 2).

If you have a complicated health history, it is not unusual for your gut to be compromised in more than one way. A common issue, for example, is an undetected virus or bacteria that can cause similar cross-reactive effects in the body.

Certain lifestyle choices may also need to be modified, including things like drinking water quality, exercise regimens, EMF exposures, etc. (See list in Chapter 2.)

NOTE: *I am also a big advocate of muscle testing to help you determine the optimal foods for yourself and/or your family. Some practitioners know how to do this. If you want to learn how to muscle test yourself, go to www.sharonharmon.com/courses for my online course Muscle Test with Confidence.*

## Look for Hidden Gluten

Many of the gluten-related grains and other suspect foods listed above are easy to spot when reading labels. However, wheat can be a little trickier. Derivatives of wheat are used in many processed foods and may be more difficult to find on a label. You also need to consider the quality and type of animal feed used when purchasing animal products.

If you are a mother working with your child and the child is still being breastfed, you need to consider what you are eating as things can pass **onto the child through breast milk**, especially if the mother's gut is also compromised. Mother-child gluten sensitivity is not uncommon.

Depending on the brand and the source, gluten-containing foods to avoid can include any of those listed below.

***Condiments, Dressings, and Sauces*** - Many condiments are thickened with gluten-containing flours and grains, and some use grain-based and/or GM corn-based vinegar as a base. GMO corn, soy, and canola oil are also often used, especially in salad dressings. Other common culprits include Worcestershire sauce, mustard, gravies, bouillon, miso, teriyaki, tamari, and soy sauce.

**Spices and Seasonings** – Spices and seasonings may contain flour-based products not obvious on the label. Natural and artificial flavors, smoke flavors, natural and artificial colors, and caramel color and flavoring can all contain gluten.

**Additives and Thickeners** – Other typical additives and thickeners that typically contain gluten include MSG, starches, vegetable gum, extenders and binders, maltodextrin, dextrin, and maltose. Another common flavor enhancer is hydrolyzed vegetable/plant protein, sometimes labeled as HVP or HPP, which can be made from wheat, corn, or soy. These additives can be found in many processed foods, including canned soups and creamed vegetables.

**Conventional Meats** – Unless chickens are fully free-range and cattle are fully pastured and "grass-fed" and "grass-finished," you need to assume they are given feed that contains a wide variety of grains and/or GMO ingredients.

Some people will be sensitive to the gluten in the meat even though it has already gone through the animal's digestive system. Consider that the animal's digestive system may also be compromised from the gluten as well as the medications they are given.

**Farm-raised Fish** – Farmed fish should be avoided as they are at least partially raised on grain and other non-marine types of food and often given medications to prevent infections that result from their containment.

They are typically raised in large penned areas that are unsanitary, so in general not healthy to eat. GM salmon, engineered to grow to full size in half the time, was approved in 2015 although not yet widely found in stores. (For more information, see this article *www.sharonharmon.com/blog/finding-quality-salmon.*)

**Pre-marinated Meats** – Meat marinade is often wheat-based. This includes store-bought turkeys and prepared hams, which are often injected with a vegetable broth that contains wheat.

**Processed Meats and Meat Substitutes** – Processed meats like beef jerky, hot dogs, sausages, bologna, pepperoni, and salami often have wheat additives, not to mention other preservatives like soy-based flavorings, nitrates, and nitrites.

Meat substitutes are often made with many of the cross-reactive ingredients listed in the last section, some highly processed with chemicals, and many suspect additives to obtain the meat-like texture and taste. Seitan is a meat substitute made from wheat.

**Conventional Milk and Eggs** – Not unlike human breast milk, any wheat/grain/GMO products fed to animals can potentially get passed through to the milk and eggs from these animals. Products made from milk, like yogurt, cheese, and ice cream, can contain additional culprit ingredients.

**Processed Cheese and Dairy Substitutes** – Cheese sprays and other processed dairy can contain wheat. Additives in shredded cheese are used to keep it from sticking together. Dairy substitutes, such as non-dairy milk creamers, can include derivatives of gluten-based products and include more suspect ingredients in general.

**Snacks** – Some manufacturers dust their fried foods, like potato chips or fries, with flour during processing, and it will not be listed on the label. Dry roasted nuts may also contain wheat not listed on the package.

**Candies and Chocolate** – Many are sweetened with barley malt, GM corn syrup, etc. Even chewing gum can contain gluten-related ingredients. If "sugar" is listed as an ingredient, assume it is made from GM beet sugar unless noted otherwise.

**Herbal Teas and Coffee Substitutes** – Some teas may have barley or barley malt added. (Rice malt is typically okay.) Some coffee substitutes are made with these as well as other grain-based ingredients. Even regular pre-ground and instant coffees can be cross-contaminated with gluten during manufacturing.

**Beer and Alcohol** – Most beers are made with barley, which is derived from wheat. There are a few beers that advertise they are gluten-free. Most alcohols are grain-based, and although the grain is distilled, it can still cause problems for some people. (Drinking beer and alcohol can also slow down the healing process because of the extra stress it puts on the liver.)

**Sprouted Breads and Grains** – It is believed that the process of sprouting grains, including wheat, changes the composition of the gluten. It does usually make it more digestible. However, I have found that sprouted bread can still affect gluten-sensitive people. This applies to sourdough bread as well.

**This may seem like a long list, but take it one category at a time**. First, improve your selection of the foods you eat most often. Chapter 5 will give you additional tips as you learn to shop gluten-free. The "cleaner" your food selections, the better results you will get when you go gluten-free.

The **key is to use fewer processed foods** and, when you do, look for those with the least number of ingredients. If you are unsure about a product or want to confirm that all ingredients are truly listed on the label, you can usually call or email the manufacturer to get more details. You can also find more specific items in my free resource, *Natural Pantry Checklist*, which you can download at *www.sharonharmon.com/freebies*.

## Food and Meal Suggestions

You may be wondering, what is there left to eat? There are still lots of great options. You want to **remove gluten and other culprit foods while maximizing your nutrition.**

The goal is to heal the digestive system and repair your "leaky gut." This, in turn, supports your immune system, reduces inflammation, and helps reduce your various symptoms. The best way to do this is by **eating plenty of unprocessed organic fruits, vegetables, legumes, nuts, and seeds as well as quality meats, fish, and eggs**, as explained in more detail in Chapter 5.

When it comes to preparing gluten-free meals, it is typically **best to cook from scratch and limit processed foods**. This may sound daunting, but once you get in the habit of doing this, you learn shortcuts.

For example, I often make larger batches of certain meals, so we can either have leftovers the next day or put the leftovers in the freezer for a quick meal on another day. This works for everything from pancakes to cooked meats, casseroles, stews, and soups.

It is not unusual for me to create a big dinner salad with lettuce and leftover meat or stir fry from the night before – just add some other cut veggies, nuts or seeds, avocado, etc., and you have a meal. You can also prepare a large salad one night and eat off of it for several days.

Some basic meal suggestions are shown below. Many I have used with my family. Use these suggestions to create your own meal plan. Begin with a week of meals and snacks, getting the ingredients in the house ahead of time, and you will start getting the hang of it.

**All the suggestions below are gluten-free, dairy-free, and GMO-free** (including no corn or soy). Also be sure to use good quality meats and eggs as well as organic products, whenever possible.

For corresponding recipes, refer to my companion gluten-free, dairy-free, and GMO-free cookbook, which you can find on my website at *www.sharonharmon.com/books*. For more ideas and brand suggestions, download my free resource, *Natural Pantry Checklist* at *www.sharonharmon.com/freebies*. (Learn more about food rotation in the next Chapter.)

### Breakfast Suggestions –

- Farm/organic boiled eggs, scrambled eggs, or omelet with veggies (You can scramble without additional liquid or use a little water instead of milk.)
- Homemade meat patty using pastured, farm-raised, organic meat with egg as a binder
- Organic turkey bacon (without nitrates or nitrites)
- Organic fruit, especially berries
- Homemade smoothie with fruit (banana, blueberries, etc.), green leafy veggie (lettuce or kale), avocado or MCT oil, and liquid base (coconut milk or ice). Play with measurements for favorite consistency and flavor. Add soaked chia seeds for more calcium or quality collagen for protein. Add

some water kefir or kombucha for a good source of natural probiotics.

- Gluten-free waffles or pancakes (It is optimal to make the batter from scratch and be sure to use the darker grade, organic maple syrup, previously called *Grade* B, because darker contains more minerals than the original *Grade* A.)
- Gluten-free toast used open-faced with nut butter, avocado, or a fried egg on top, using ghee instead of butter
- Homemade gluten-free muffins (Store-bought are not very nutritious, and most have questionable ingredients. Find recipes online or in my companion cookbook available at *www.sharonharmon.com/books*.)
- Organic coconut or cashew-based yogurt topped with nuts, fruit, and/or chia seeds, or a nut/seed-based granola (Plain or vanilla is best as fruit flavors usually have more additives. Homemade yogurt is optimal.)
- Some can tolerate "gluten-free oatmeal" if soaked overnight and drained before cooking in the morning, since soaking helps to break down the phytic acid for easier digestion (Make sure it is produced in a gluten-free factory or use groats), topped with fruit, chia seeds, nuts, and/or dairy-free yogurt

You may have noticed that I did not include non-dairy "milk" products as these often contain questionable ingredients: emulsifiers, sweeteners, fortified (man-made) vitamins, and other additives. If you need a milk source to eat a healthy gluten-free granola, for example, it is best to make your own.

You can make it fresh by simply blending a handful of raw nuts in a few cups of water using a blender and pouring it through a strainer. Cashew milk is my favorite. Quality coconut milk is another option.

### Lunch/Dinner Suggestions –

- Grass-fed/pastured meats such as beef, buffalo/bison, lamb, etc. (You can find good local sources at *www.localharvest.org*.)
- Burgers made from ground grass-fed pastured meats served between lettuce leaves or quality gluten-free rolls or on top of a salad
- Pastured/GMO-free feed poultry, such as roast chicken, turkey legs, etc.
- Homemade chicken nuggets, using good quality chicken and almond meal or rice flour instead of breadcrumbs
- Brown rice or quinoa cooked in homemade bone broth, using bones left over from roasted chicken and other quality meats (Find recipes online or in my companion cookbook available at *www.sharonharmon.com/books*.)
- Homemade soups and stews, another way to use bone broth
- Green salads with multiple vegetables, avocado, nuts/seeds, etc., add ground flax seed for extra texture (no croutons) and homemade dressing with non-grain-based vinegar (see below)
- Pasta dishes, like spaghetti, using gluten-free organic brown rice pasta (Watch out for quinoa pasta since many include corn.)

- Steamed or baked vegetables topped with avocado or coconut oil and quality salt
- Stir fry using coconut oil, a variety of chopped vegetables, shredded meat, and cooked rice or quinoa
- Baked sweet potato topped with steamed vegetables and sea salt and ghee (or quality butter if you can tolerate it)
- Homemade fries from sliced red potato or sweet potato and coconut oil with salt
- Organic lunch meats like chicken or turkey breast rolled up with lettuce, tomato, and avocado, with or without a coconut or rice-based wrap

Salad dressings are one of the hardest foods to find "clean" without preservatives, GM ingredients, unhealthy seed oils, etc. Instead, it is best to make your own. An easy base salad dressing uses proportions of 1/3 apple cider vinegar and 2/3 quality olive oil with sea salt and spices of choice. Shake or blend well for a creamier consistency.

## *Snack Suggestions* –

- Organic hummus with cut-up veggies (cucumber, carrot, celery, broccoli, bell pepper, etc.)
- Cherry tomatoes
- Celery sticks or apple slices with nut or seed butter
- Fruit bowl using fresh fruit
- Baked apple with a little honey and cinnamon sprinkled on top
- Homemade carrot or kale chips (Find recipes online.)
- Roasted seaweed snacks (Make sure not made with canola oil.)

- Rice cakes (preferably brown rice) with nut butter or egg salad
- Bean or casava-based chips (without corn) with dairy-free guacamole, organic hummus, or naturally fermented sauerkraut
- Roasted chickpeas
- Naturally fermented (without vinegar) veggies, pickles, carrot sticks, etc.
- Gluten-free (and corn-free) crackers with nut butter
- Frozen popsicles made from leftover smoothies (see above)
- Frozen grapes, peas, or carrots
- Gluten-free, plain potato chips made with avocado or olive oil (without flour coating or canola/seed oils)
- Black olives in quality olive oil
- Half of an avocado eaten with sea salt and a spoon
- Gluten-free and soy-free beef or turkey jerky
- Handful of sprouted seeds or raw nuts (nuts preferably soaked to reduce phytic acid)
- Homemade trail mix with raw cashews, pumpkin or sunflower seeds, coconut strips, and cranberries or raisins

**The goal is to replace all your gluten-containing foods with healthy alternatives, not a bunch of gluten-free junk foods, which are now abundant in stores**. Limit overly processed foods and avoid products with preservatives. Even chips and rice cakes, which are more processed, should be eaten in moderation. You want to supply the body with more nutrition for healing.

Just because something says "gluten-free" does not mean it is good for you as it can still contain suspect ingredients. It is critical to read ingredient lists and not blindly trust "gluten-free" labeled products. Many gluten-free breads, for example, contain soy, corn, and/or canola (all GM crops), including xanthan gum, which is often made from corn.

Ultimately, you want to work toward eating organic, locally grown veggies and fruits and good quality meats/eggs from animals that are pastured/free-range and not fed or finished with grains. All of these foods are naturally gluten-free.

**If this is new to you, start with baby steps.** First, work on the gluten and your "culprit" foods. Then consciously reduce GMO-based ingredients. Over time, especially as you start to feel better, you will want to continue to make improvements. Eventually, you may want to start your own garden!

The next chapter will explore where some people get stuck or unknowingly create another health-related issue. I will also give you suggestions for the best ways to eat out gluten-free and negotiate meals with family and friends.

## Chapter 3 Summary

∞ Not all gluten-free products are equal. Just because something is labeled gluten-free does not mean it is healthy. You need to be selective and know that other foods can mimic the effects of gluten.

∞ Many gluten-free products have questionable additives or less nutritious ingredients that can be "cross-reactive." You also need to be concerned about GMO-based ingredients.

∞ Knowing which products and ingredients to substitute before you start your gluten-free journey increases follow-through. Review the grain options once more and use the meal suggestions in this chapter to get prepared.

∞ Consider your kitchen and how you prepare your food before getting started as cross-contamination can happen between gluten-based foods and gluten-free foods. If working with one person in the family, consider making the whole family gluten-free. If not, create separate prep areas in your kitchen.

∞ The most common cross-reactive foods include oats, soy, corn, and other genetically modified (GM) crops and cow's milk dairy. Other foods may be cross-reactive for certain people (see list in Chapter 3) depending on your health status and how much healing needs to occur. For more challenging health issues, working with a knowledgeable holistic health practitioner can be beneficial.

∞ Gluten can be hidden in mother's breast milk as well as many processed foods like condiments, dressings, and additives, as well as certain meats and meat substitutes, dairy and dairy substitutes, treats, drinks, etc. (See extensive list in Chapter 3.)

∞ Many meal suggestions free of gluten, dairy, and GMOs are listed in the chapter. The key is to replace gluten-based foods with healthy alternatives like organic fruits, vegetables, legumes, nuts/seeds, and quality animal products while limiting processed and packaged foods.

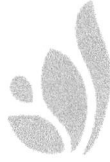

## CHAPTER 4

# More Gluten Considerations

Some of you may be ready to jump right in. Others may want to experiment and discover which gluten-free options are best, especially for children, before removing and/or replacing too many existing foods.

Remember, however, that certain cravings and food addictions will not dissipate until all sources of gluten and related foods are removed. For children who are especially picky eaters, it will be important to remove gluten and dairy/casein from the diet at the same time, due to similar reactions in the body, as explained in Chapter 1.

**To get the most out of going gluten-free and doing it the right way, you need to understand additional concepts** that will be explained in this chapter.

In previous chapters, you learned that you need to be very selective when purchasing gluten-free products. They are not all created equal. Yet, you need to be conscious of not narrowing down your food choices too much. (In Chapter 5 you will learn additional tips for shopping gluten-free.)

This chapter will explain why food rotation is important and what to look for in other products you use in your home and on your body. Also included are tips to negotiate eating out in restaurants and eating meals with family and friends. (Chapter 6 explains how to bake gluten-free.)

Knowing this information before you start your journey can make all the difference.

## Importance of Food Rotation

As you start including gluten-free food options in your diet, **consider how often you are eating the same thing**.

For example, rice is an easy substitute for wheat in gluten-free products. Before you know it, you are eating cooked rice, rice pasta, rice milk, rice cakes, rice crackers, etc. Instead, it is better to rotate the gluten-free grains you are using. Go back to Chapter 3 to see the list.

Too much of any food group has the **potential to create health problems**. More common examples include the following.

***Becoming Sensitive to a New Food Group*** – Using a variety and rotating natural gluten substitutes, especially gluten-free grains, prevents your body from becoming reactive to a new food as the key to eating healthy is to eat a variety of foods and/or food groups.

As I mentioned above, you may find that you are eating rice at every meal. Your digestive system needs variety. Some of your gluten-free substitutes should be made with other gluten-free grain sources such as amaranth, buckwheat, millet, quinoa, sorghum, and grain-free options. (More about this in Chapter 6.)

**Creating a Nutrient Deficiency** – When you limit certain foods like gluten and dairy, it is tempting to find alternative foods that you like and stick to those, especially packaged foods. In addition to creating a possible sensitivity, you need to consider how nutrient-dense these products are. Many are not much better than eating white bread, which has little nutritious value or fiber.

Instead, be sure to include an assortment of gluten-free grains and a good variety of other foods, like vegetables, nuts, meats, fats, and fruits, which gives your body a better balance of nutrients. You want to obtain as many nutrients as possible from your food. However, you may also need to add supplements as you could already be nutrient deficient from your gluten sensitivities, as I explained in previous chapters.

**Becoming Food Toxic** – Some gluten substitutes are healthier than others. Nut flour is a common example. It is good in moderation, but it is found in many baked goods. Nut flours go rancid easily, and I am not convinced the oils in the nut flours are meant to be eaten after being heated at high temperatures.

Almond flour, for instance, is used in many baked goods including crackers. Another common ingredient is xanthan gum, which is often made from GM corn and can be a gut irritant for some people. (See a more comprehensive list of ingredients to avoid in Chapters 3 and 5.)

**Creating an Oxalate Toxicity** – Oxalate is a naturally occurring molecule that may appear as sharp crystals in different parts of the body. Oxalates are found in many foods but are highest in spinach, nuts (especially almonds and peanuts), and several other more natural foods as well as certain fruits and vegetables.

When going gluten-free, you will find almond flour/meal in many packaged foods, for example, as a substitute for gluten-containing grains and dairy products. This adds up quickly, especially if you are also eating nuts and baking with an almond meal. (Nuts are meant to be eaten in limited amounts and preferably in their whole, raw form after soaking. Seeds have less oxalates.)

Ironically, gluten-free grains like amaranth, buckwheat, and quinoa are also higher in oxalates and best used after soaking and dumping the water. Oxalate symptoms vary with each person, as they affect your mitochondria, which are present in every system of the body. Some people are more sensitive than others. (To learn more about oxalates, see Sally Norton's book *Toxic Superfoods*.)

I can relate to the list above, because **I unknowingly did all of it incorrectly when we first started** eating gluten-free. And, since I was one of the early adopters of eating gluten-free, we learned some lessons the hard way.

At first, we ate rice everything. Then, after finding out how good almond flour tasted in my recipes, I added it to everything that needed flour or breadcrumbs until I learned about oxalates a few years later.

I had created a new problem in my body.

Turns out that I had several oxalate symptoms and had to systematically cut back on the high-oxalate foods my family and I were eating. (Reducing oxalates must be done slowly, see Norton's book or work with a knowledgeable practitioner who understands oxalates.)

**Optimally, you want to rotate certain foods daily so that you have variety**. Think of the different food groups that you typically eat, like grains, veggies, fruit, meat, fats, etc., and consider selecting a different option from each for every meal, while you continue to avoid gluten (and dairy). Begin by trying not to eat the same thing two days in a row and work from there. Ultimately, you will find what works best for you and/or your family.

NOTE: *I am also a big advocate of muscle testing to help you determine the optimal foods for yourself and/or your family. Some practitioners know how to do this. If you want to learn how to muscle test yourself, go to www.sharonharmon.com/courses for my online course* Muscle Test with Confidence.

## Gluten in Other Products

Did you know that gluten can be found in body products, vitamins and other supplements, pharmaceuticals, and a few other unlikely places? If you are gluten-sensitive, you will want to read the ingredients in everything you purchase.

This includes your **bath and body products**, especially since your skin is an extension of your digestive system. You will want to look at the ingredients in soaps and shampoos, skin lotions, cosmetics, lipsticks, sunscreens, nail polish, toothpaste, hand sanitizers, etc.

The skin is considered your largest organ and what you put on it can get absorbed "transdermally" through the skin into your bloodstream as well as lymph nodes and fascia. Some molecules in body products may be too large to be fully absorbed, but as more products use nanotechnology, molecules are getting smaller, allowing more and deeper penetration.

This is not good if the ingredients are not optimal. It is possible to react more strongly to a body product than a food because it bypasses your digestive system.

So, when you are gluten-sensitive, you do not want your body products to contain gluten, or other toxic ingredients for that matter.

Unfortunately, body products are not well-regulated. In the United States, for example, the Food and Drug Administration (FDA) has banned very few ingredients from being used in bath and body products, including cosmetics.

Rather, it is the companies that make and market the products that have the responsibility to ensure their safety. Ingredients labeled as "other ingredients" or "fragrance" could encompass a wide variety of undisclosed ingredients.

A common body product ingredient is hydrolyzed wheat protein. There could be other gluten-containing derivatives as well, such as starch, dextrate, maltose, etc. It is best to look for products that say "gluten-free" on the package or, even better, "gluten-free verified."

Something that says "no gluten added" is not good enough, as that means they did not add gluten; however, one of the ingredients may inherently contain gluten. You also need to consider cross-reactive ingredients, as explained in Chapter 3. (You can find gluten-free certified body products in a database created by Gluten-Free Certification Organization or GFCO at *www.gfco.org*.)

If you are taking **supplements, such as vitamins and minerals, or pharmaceuticals,** you will want to check their ingredients as well. Many include fillers (or excipients) that could contain gluten or derivatives of GM corn or soy. The coating on a pill may also contain these ingredients (as well as food dyes).

Examples include:

- Starch or cross-linked starch
- Dextrate
- Cyclodextrin

- Dextrin or dextrimaltose (may be extracted from barley malt)
- Maltose or maltodextrin (can be extracted from wheat or corn)
- Pregelatinized starch
- Sodium starch glycolate
- Caramel color

It has also been found that certain prescription medications can create what seems like gluten sensitivity in some people. So, if you have not had good results with a gluten-free diet in the past, you may need to consider the side effects of the medication(s) you are taking.

Certain **whole food supplements** that contain grasses can be an issue, such as wheat grass and barley grass. These are often found in "green" powders and supplements. Although not technically a grain when still in grass form, these greens can cause problems for some people.

**Other unlikely places** to find gluten include:

- Storebought playdough (You can find homemade recipes for playdough online. Just make it with rice flour instead of basic white flour.)
- Non-adhesive envelops or stamps (ones that you lick to seal)
- Braces and other orthodontic materials, especially the plastic components
- Adhesive bandages or medical tape (If you use them regularly, you should check those too.)

Don't forget your pets. **Commercial pet foods** often contain grains and GMO ingredients. Not only are these ingredients bad for your pets, as many are not traditionally grain eaters, but you can be exposed to gluten when handling the pet food. At a minimum, make sure your pet's food and treats are gluten-free.

## Eating with Family and Friends

Eating gluten-free away from home can be a challenge. Let's first consider some options when you plan to eat a meal at a family member's or a friend's house. Honestly, it is easier to meet at a restaurant where you can freely ask questions of your server as well as pick and choose what you want (as explained in the next section). You may want to suggest this as an alternative.

However, if you are going to eat at someone's house, I find it is best to **let them know ahead of time** that you would love to attend, and that you are currently eating gluten-free.

If they ask you how they can accommodate you, great. Give them a few ideas like you can't have anything made with bread or typical flour, no croutons in the salad, or no pasta. If you have also eliminated dairy (specifically milk, cheese, and yogurt), you should let them know that as well.

You can ask about the meal and provide suggestions. For example, if your host is having spaghetti, the meatballs can be made without breadcrumbs (or with almond flour instead of breadcrumbs); the pasta can be made with rice noodles (which are the easiest gluten-free option to cook); and ask that parmesan cheese be left on the side. If it was me, I would offer to bring the noodles as well as some gluten-free rolls to share.

Unfortunately, not everyone will be that accommodating. Some will find it overwhelming. Others don't understand how detrimental gluten can be to your health or are uncomfortable with changing how they make their meals.

It can also be awkward to keep asking, "What is in this?" as food is being passed around the table. That is why it is optimal to have an open discussion before the event occurs.

Of course, if you are more gluten-sensitive or going through a strict phase of no gluten, the above scenario may not be optimal. The host's kitchen is likely not gluten-free, and you need to **consider cross-contamination**. Gluten-based foods prepared on cutting boards, countertops, toaster and oven racks, etc. can leave gluten residue that can potentially contaminate your gluten-free food. (See more about cross-contamination in the next section.)

I have found over the years it is **easiest to bring food** to both share with others and have as a backup for myself and my family. Most conventional turkeys, for example, are basted with liquids that contain gluten. So, at Thanksgiving, I might bring a big green salad to share, an avocado, some nuts or seeds, and a cooked turkey breast so I can make a hearty salad if there ends up being little I can eat. (I typically also bring my homemade salad dressing and quality salt.)

Once in a great while, I do eat gluten on purpose as I did one Thanksgiving. (Get the details about me "getting glutened" in my article at *www.sharonharmon.com/blog/getting-glutened*.) It can be hard to resist some of your favorite foods. And, who does not love a traditional Thanksgiving dinner with all the fixings?

So, maybe once every year or two, I give myself permission to "go all out" for two reasons: (1) I can eat like everyone else and enjoy my favorite childhood foods and (2) I can see how I react as some people can be less strict over time as they heal their gut. I might regret it the next day, as I do not feel optimal, but it helps me keep tabs on my body and be more selective going forward.

(I would not suggest doing this early in your gluten-free process, as it takes a while to get rid of the gliadin antibodies once again. And definitely not, if you are extremely gluten-sensitive or have Celiac Disease.)

## Eating at Restaurants

When eating at a restaurant, the first thing to consider is the type of establishment. Although some fast-food restaurants now offer gluten-free items on their menu, the substitute ingredients can still be questionable. If you do find yourself in this situation, it is best to **ask for the list of ingredients**.

For example, if they offer gluten-free bread, ask to see the package. If they offer gluten-free pizza, ask for a list of the ingredients used in the pizza crust. Typically, you will still find GMO ingredients like corn, soy, and canola oil listed.

It is often better to eat in a nicer restaurant where meals are made from scratch. You can **ask specific questions** of your server who can talk to the chef if necessary. It is also more likely that certain menu items can be modified to be gluten-free.

Over time, you will find the restaurants that best suit your dietary needs.

Some things to consider or ask about include:

- A separate surface should be used to prepare their gluten-free meals so there is no cross-contamination. (At home, a clean plate can be used.)
- Certain thickeners used in salad dressings and marinades can include gluten. (That is why I usually bring my homemade salad dressing when we eat out.)

- Flour is often used as a base for soups and sauces and this flour can contain gluten. Soy sauces also typically contain gluten.
- The oils used to fry foods can be used multiple times for breaded and non-breaded items, causing cross-contamination. If eating French fries, ask if they are cooked in a separate fryer and make sure the fries are not dusted with flour.
- Marinated meat seasonings often contain textured vegetable protein (TVP), which may contain gluten. Some restaurants may also cook meat using a hydrolyzed vegetable protein (HVP), which could contain gluten.
- If non-dairy products, such as creamer or whipped cream, are used some ingredients may be questionable.
- Wheat and/or barley are often used to make soy products such as tempeh or seitan, both of which can be used in oriental dishes.
- Flavored rice and other side dishes like hash browns may contain wheat products.
- Flour is sometimes added to sushi rice to make it stickier or French fries to make them less greasy.

Until proven otherwise, you should always **assume your server is not gluten-literate**. There are many times a server has told me, "Yes, that is gluten-free," but if I ask the question differently or ask for more details, I find out it is not. You can't expect a server to know as much as you do. Plus the server may have no idea how detrimental gluten can be.

If necessary, ask to see an ingredient list or to speak directly to the chef.

You should also confirm your special order is correct when it arrives, especially if something looks suspect.

The person in the kitchen may automatically add cheese and croutons to your salad, for example, since that is what they are used to. And, be sure to refuse the complimentary bread when offered, so you are not tempted.

Often, one of the safest meals to eat is steamed vegetables and a piece of meat (or a baked potato). I often get a large salad with baked chicken (not breaded, using salt and pepper only), asking them to eliminate the croutons, cheese, and salad dressing. Then ask for olive oil and wine or balsamic vinegar instead (since regular vinegar is typically made from GM corn).

I often bring a homemade salad dressing with me. It may feel uncomfortable the first time, but you can make it inconspicuous, by using a small jar. (It also depends if you are eating with close family/friends or trying to impress a new client or significant other.)

As we move on to learn the optimal ways to shop and bake gluten-free, keep in mind what was discussed in the first few chapters.

You have learned so much about the right ways and the wrong ways to eat gluten-free. Most importantly, how removing dairy and GM foods can take a gluten-free diet to a whole new level.

The next chapter will be a great resource for you, because the "cleaner" you shop for food (and other gluten-containing products), the easier it is to eat healthy.

# Chapter 4 Summary

∞ When eating gluten-free (and dairy-free), you need to be cautious about how often you eat the same substitutes so you do not become sensitive to another food group.

∞ Eating too limited for a long period can potentially create nutrient deficiencies.

∞ Food toxicity can potentially occur if you eat an abundance of the same food. Some foods, like nuts, are made to eat in limited quantities and more like a snack, so be careful how much nut milk and nut flour you consume.

∞ Other ingredients often used in gluten-free products, like xanthan gum (and even guar gum), can be problematic for some people.

∞ Oxalate toxicity can also occur over time if your substitute foods are continuously high in oxalates, like nuts and spinach as well as other grains and vegetables.

∞ Optimally, you want to rotate foods daily so you have a variety from different food groups like vegetables, fruit, grains, nuts/seeds, animal products, fats, etc. You will obtain a wider spectrum of nutrients as well.

∞ Bath and body products can also include gluten-based ingredients, which can get absorbed into the body through the skin. Read the ingredients carefully.

∞ Medications and natural supplements can also contain gluten, dairy, as well as GMO-based ingredients or derivatives, especially in added fillers and coatings. (See partial list in Chapter 4.)

∞ Other unlikely hidden sources of gluten include playdough, lickable seals, dental materials, plastics, bandages, and pet food.

∞ Eating with friends and family is easier if you plan. Talk to your host ahead of time and bring food to share.

∞ Eating at a restaurant can be a challenge, but if you research your options online before heading out, it can be an easier experience. Making sure your server truly understands what gluten-free (and dairy-free) means is also important. (See Chapter 4 for additional tips.)

# CHAPTER 5

# Shopping Gluten-free

People often ask me what I purchase when I go grocery shopping, knowing that I feel better eating gluten-free. I tend to shop at multiple locations. We are fortunate to have several more natural options like Whole Foods, Trader Joe's, and Sprouts, as well as multiple conventional grocery stores in our area.

However, no matter where I shop, I am very selective.

**Not all "health food" products are created equal**, even if you shop at a "natural food store." You have to look at ingredient lists and know your products. **You also need to know your containers**. For example, I stopped purchasing a good brand of almond butter years ago because they switched the containers from glass to plastic, and I know that greasy foods absorb the chemicals in the plastic.

If you and/or your family eat gluten-free, there are additional things to watch out for when food shopping. This chapter will reinforce what you have already learned: Many gluten-free products are not that healthy. Various additives and suspect ingredients are used to make them taste better.

Certain gluten-free grains have their drawbacks as well and can cause additional issues, some of which I covered in Chapter 4.

First, I will explain what to look for when shopping, so you know what not to purchase. This will help to narrow down your selections. Then I will list some of my favorite gluten-free options. They might not all be what I call "perfect," but the lists will give you ideas of what to purchase for yourself and/or your family so you can eat gluten-free the right way.

*Caution for extra sensitive people*: *The industry standard for "gluten-free" products allows them to contain up to 20 parts per million (ppm) of gluten. If you have celiac disease or you are severely sensitive to gluten, you may need to shop for other gluten-free brands (ones that are produced in a gluten-free facility). Call the manufacturer if you need clarification.*

# What NOT to Buy

So, before I tell you what I normally purchase, I need to tell you **what I do not purchase**.

It is more than just eliminating your typical junk foods. Yes, you want to eliminate gluten, dairy and GMOs, but you also want to eliminate potentially toxic foods that could make your food sensitivity worse. You need to consider how the food is grown, how it is prepared, the added ingredients, as well as the containers and packaging of the food.

As a general rule, I typically *do not buy* the following types of products, no matter where I shop.

***Oils and Greasy Products in Plastic Containers*** – Greasy and fatty foods tend to absorb the chemicals found in plastic, and when we eat these foods, the chemicals end up in our bodies. Examples include bisphenol A (BPA) and its newer cousin bisphenol S (BPS). However, plastics contain many chemicals we have yet to hear about.

So, you need to limit foods like nut butters, vegetable oils, meats, cheese, or other greasy-type foods in plastic bottles, cans (or tetra packs) with plastic liners, or plastic wrap. You should not store these foods in plastic bags or containers at home either. Use glass instead.

***Genetically Modified (or GMO) Ingredients*** – Unfortunately, this rules out many packaged food options in all grocery stores, including health food stores. So many "healthy" processed foods have corn, soy, canola, and even cottonseed oil in their ingredient list, and it is estimated that 85% to 95% of these GMO foods are genetically modified.

Corn, for example, is added to all sorts of foods under many different names. Additives are often derived from corn. A few common examples include ascorbic acid (Vitamin C), citrate, maltodextrin, MSG, natural flavors, and many fake sugars (see below). The list is extensive. (A good list can be found at *www.livecornfree.com.*)

Other GM ingredients to stay away from include: beet sugar, alfalfa, certain papaya, crookneck squash, and some zucchini. If it does not state the sugar as "cane sugar", you need to assume it is GM beet sugar.

***Gluten-free (GF) Prepackaged Products*** – Check all ingredients in prepackaged foods that state they are gluten-free. Many packaged gluten-free foods are just not healthy, including those at health food stores. Some are glorified junk food, with plenty of sugar to make up for the lack of gluten.

Others have additional suspect ingredients like GMOs (see above), oatmeal (which you should stay away from if you are strictly GF), unhealthy binders such as carrageenan (a known stomach irritant) and xanthan gum (often corn-derived), etc. Unfortunately, this includes most breads, cereals, crackers, and cookies. Be selective.

*Artificial and GMO Sugars* - Many gluten-free products contain extra sweeteners to make up for what may seem like lack of taste. If an ingredient is listed as "sugar", assume that it is genetically modified, as beet sugar is now a GM crop and the least expensive to use. For it to be non-GMO, the label should read non-GM sugar, organic sugar, turbinado sugar, or some other sugar specifically not beet sugar.

If you are already eating more naturally, you likely know to avoid "fake sugars" like aspartame and saccharin. However, with the introduction of "low-glycemic foods" there are many more man-made, highly processed sugars I would advise avoiding as they are devoid of nutrients and/or can negatively affect the gut. And, many are derived from GM corn. More common ones include ethanol, mannitol, sorbitol, sucralose, and xylitol. (See *www.livecornfree.com* for more.)

*Prechopped and Prewashed Produce* - I do buy this type of produce when nothing else is available, but only if it is organic. However, many prewashed items such as lettuce, kale, and other chopped vegetables are washed in a bath with one or more chemicals, even organic varieties. Baby carrots, for example, are known to be washed in a chlorine bath. Fruits and vegetables also start to lose nutrients the moment they are peeled and cut. It may be more convenient, but it is less nutritious.

*Salad Dressings, Dips, Sauces, and Hummus* - The number one reason to avoid these premade and packaged foods is that most of them contain canola, soy, corn, or cottonseed oil (all genetically modified crops), or a seed and/or vegetable oil. If you do find a product that is free of GM ingredients and other suspect "natural" ingredients, be sure to recheck the ingredient list once in a while.

I was buying quality organic hummus, for example, until I realized that they changed the olive oil to canola oil after being out of stock for a while. This can happen to any grocery product as manufacturers find ways to cut costs and/or larger manufacturers purchase smaller organic companies. (Also consider the container as greasy foods will leach the plastic. Glass is better.)

**Fruit Juices** – You should avoid these in general. Drinking fruit juice unnecessarily spikes your blood sugar. Prepackaged juices are also typically made from concentrate and/or have been pasteurized so it has little nutritional value. Some fruit drinks contain added colorants and more recently have been found to contain heavy metals such as lead and arsenic. We use it for special occasions only.

This is the same for many coconut water drinks as well – most are pasteurized and some have added sweeteners. (To wean your child off fruit juice, cut it with water and increase the percentage of water over time. Use cold mint tea or fruity-flavored teas like hibiscus instead.)

**Sparkling Drinks and Kombucha** – As a general rule, you should stay away from soft drinks as they contain way too much sugar and other suspect ingredients. Many people turn to fruit-flavored sparkling drinks (or fruit energy drinks) instead.

However, you should know most brands use "natural flavors" rather than real fruit juice to create the fruit flavor. These natural flavors can be created using many suspect ingredients including those derived from GM corn as mentioned earlier.

Homemade kombucha can be beneficial for some people and is preferred over store-bought varieties, as these can contain added sweeteners and colorants so select carefully. (Fermented drinks and foods can leach plastic so they are best in glass bottles.)

***Fortified Products*** - You should stay away from fortified products in general. Theoretically, packaged foods with added vitamins may sound like a good thing. The problem is that most of these vitamins are synthetically derived and not readily used by the body.

For example, added vitamin D is usually D2 (man-made), and not D3, which is what your body really needs. Folic acid is another synthetic nutrient that actually harms the body, which needs the natural version, called folate. (Learn more about folate at *www.chriskresser.com/folate-vs-folic-acid.*)

***Fake Meats and Cheese*** - I mentioned farmed-raised fish and meat substitutes in Chapter 3. Neither provides much nutritional value and may actually be hurting you. The same with cheese substitutes, or what I tend to call fake cheese. These are additional food categories I avoid.

Store-bought fake meats and cheese typically fall into the category of ultra-processed food, which are foods made of substances extracted from other foods, often using chemicals. Plus many suspect ingredients are added to give the fake meat or cheese the taste and consistency of the real thing. Essentially, they are man-made foods, which I try to avoid as much as possible.

After reading the list above, **you may be asking yourself, "What is there left to buy?" Believe it or not, there is still quite a list** of items. Not everyone will immediately cut out all the culprit foods listed above.

However, if you want to be healthy, you must educate yourself. There may be other ingredients to consider as well, such as "natural flavors," which can be used to mean many different things, and "low-fat" or "low-sugar," which often means the product has alternative, unhealthy ingredients.

## My Favorite Grocery Items

So, what do I purchase when I go grocery shopping? I **typically buy organic as well as grass-fed, pastured, and wild-caught** when it comes to animal products. I also like to purchase products as close to their **naturally-grown state as possible**. When purchasing processed foods, I like products with the **least number of ingredients**, and all the ingredients must be names that I recognize as food (not a chemical derivative or preservative).

**Below I give you some general guidance**. I suggest also reviewing the hidden sources of gluten as explained and listed in Chapter 3. And, you can find more specific items and brands by downloading my free resource, *Natural Pantry Checklist*, from my website at *www.sharonharmon.com/freebies*.

*Produce* – As I mentioned earlier, I prefer to have something fresher that is still intact. Plus, prewashed and prepackaged produce is more expensive and does not typically last very long in the refrigerator.

When I can, I shop for produce at a farmer's market. If you have a health food store nearby, you will likely find more organic options there. Other grocery stores vary greatly depending on the chain as well as the location. We have one local chain of stores that has a great organic produce selection in one part of town but minimal in another. (It depends on interest, so ask your store managers for more options.)

A few things I get regularly include: lettuce, dino kale, celery, radishes, broccoli, cucumber, avocado, whole carrots, onions, red potatoes, lemons, apples, bananas, pears, raspberries, grapes, and other items in season. (Learn which high-pesticide crops to avoid at *www.sharonharmon.com/blog/know-your-pesticides.*)

**Meats and Eggs** – Optimally, I try to get our meats and eggs from local farmers I trust. Some grocery stores offer better meat options in their frozen section, but you must read the labels as wording can be tricky. Look for beef that is grass-fed and finished, chicken and eggs that are pastured and given GMO-free feed, etc. Compare several brands to find the best option.

Even better are meats (and eggs) labeled with "no hormones" and "no antibiotics," since both are often used in conventional meats. Optimally, you would want "no vaccines" on the label as well, but this is very difficult to find, even from local farmers. Meats are usually flash frozen, so I do not worry about the plastic wrapping, and I remove the plastic to defrost.

I do sometimes purchase uncured, organic beef hot dogs and/or lunch meat. However, I prefer to go to a butcher who typically has better, less processed options (and I ask them to wrap it in paper). (If chicken eggs are an issue, consider duck or quail eggs.)

**Fish** – Another great frozen item is fish, especially Sockeye wild-caught salmon. Or, you can wait until wild salmon is in season (usually August in the United States) and stock up. I usually have the butcher cut large slabs to meal sizes for my family and individually freeze them in freezer bags with wax paper. (The butcher will remove the skin and bones for you.)

Fish labeled as "wild-caught" is key, especially salmon, since genetically modified (GM) salmon was approved in 2015. There are a few GM salmon farms in operation, but it is rarely found in stores yet. (It is not required to be labeled.) "Wild-caught" also helps you avoid farmed fish, since they are typically fed GM grains. (More in Chapter 3.)

Quality canned fish is another option. A good tip I learned is that canned fish has to be wild-caught because farmed fish does not can well. I look for wild Alaskan or Sockeye salmon, which is great for cold salmon salad, as well as canned sardines, optimally in water without salt. (Avoid any canned fish in cans with plastic liners.)

**Frozen** – Be wary of any prepackaged and prepared frozen items that have added flavors and sauces, such as prepared stir-fries, as these often have suspect ingredients. Instead, it is best to find single-ingredient frozen products like organic fruits (which are great for smoothies) and organic vegetables (which work good in soups and homemade stir-fries).

When you need to use some convenient foods, such as frozen gluten-free pizza crusts, waffles, or fries, it is best to read the ingredients in all the available options so you can select the "cleanest" version and one without your culprit ingredients.

**Nuts and Seeds** – It can be difficult to find organic nuts and seeds, so I at least make sure they are raw and unsalted. However, you need to be aware that some nuts are allowed to be modified and still be called raw.

For example, since 2007 the U.S. Department of Agriculture (USDA) has required all "raw" almonds sold in the United States to be chemically treated, irradiated, or pasteurized (steamed), yet they can be labeled as raw. I no longer purchase conventional raw almonds, almond butter, or almond flour. (The only place to purchase truly "raw" almonds is direct from a farmer or through a company with a waiver to sell in small quantities.)

Most "raw" cashews also go through a high-temperature process to ensure the toxic resin inherent in the shell is not released during the shelling process. I like to get a variety of nuts as well as sunflower and pumpkin seeds, as seeds have fewer oxalates than nuts. (See Chapter 4.) You can also usually find organic chia seeds and hemp seeds.

**Grains** – There are not many prepackaged products that are gluten-free, oat-free, GMO-free and organic. If you also limit the amounts of almond meal you consume, that leaves few options.

Additionally, most store-bought gluten-free breads include xanthan gum as the substitute for the fluffiness that gluten provides. I will sometimes get bread with xanthan gum to use maybe once a week or a couple of times a month, but I suggest not using it daily. Even better, find home-baked gluten-free bread at a local farmer's market.

I typically avoid most grocery store gluten-free crackers and cookies as well, for the reasons discussed earlier in this chapter. Another option is to get plain rice cakes, which can be used instead of bread with some toppings. Other grain-based products that I purchase include brown rice, basmati rice, quinoa, brown rice spaghetti pasta (with minimal ingredients), all of which are inherently gluten-free.

**Dairy** – If you eat dairy, raw would be best, as organic dairy is often heated at high temperatures, which gives little nutritional value. However, organic (and minimally processed) is better than the alternative. Conventional milk and milk products are from animals fed with GM grains and given pharmaceuticals.

You also need to consider the packaging because most dairy comes in plastic, which leaches into the dairy over time. When purchasing butter, purchase sticks wrapped in wax paper, when possible, as the foil wrappers can contain non-stick chemicals. I look for cultured and grass-fed butter.

If dairy-free, use ghee instead of butter. When it comes to other dairy substitutes, I typically stick to coconut milk as organic brands with few ingredients are usually easy to find. Be sure to read the ingredients closely on all other dairy substitutes and avoid fortified versions.

Other items I purchase regularly include:

- Organic beef or turkey jerky (flavored with salt and pepper only)
- Organic virgin coconut oil
- Organic virgin olive oil (from a trusted source as most olive oils are mixed with cheaper vegetable oils unless purchased directly from a farm)
- Organic dried cranberries and raisins (free of nitrates, good for trail mixes)
- Organic herb teas (great as cold drinks in the summer, be careful of tea bags that use plastic)
- Organic maple syrup (darker color for more nutrients)

## When You Need a Treat

There are **a few products I purchase once in a while, either as a treat or for special occasions**.

It might be best to avoid these items in the beginning of your healing journey. However, if you decide to continue eating gluten-free, and hopefully GMO-free too, you need to have some options. (Even in more healthy sources, xanthan gum is one ingredient that is difficult to always avoid.)

Here are some suggestions:

- Organic coconut water (unpasteurized when possible, not from concentrate)
- Sparkling natural mineral water (most flavored varieties do not use real fruit juice)
- Natural ginger ale (made with minimal ingredients and real ginger)
- Snack bars with minimal ingredients (typically nut or seed-based)
- Gluten-free pie crust (without xanthan gum if possible)
- Dark or semi-sweet chocolate bar or chips (without milk or soy lecithin, look for one with minimal ingredients)
- Organic gluten and corn-free pizza crust (without xanthan gum if possible) to make homemade pizza with tomato sauce and veggies (no cheese)
- Organic fruit spread thickened with pectin and slightly sweetened (great alternative to maple syrup on pancakes and crepes)
- Organic potato chips made with coconut or avocado oil and salt
- Bean, casava, or lentil chips (in lieu of corn chips) for dipping
- Macadamia nuts or cashews, dry roasted and salted

Where we live, we are fortunate to have several healthier grocery store options and many farmer's markets to choose from, with farmers who are very conscientious of the food they grow and raise. **You may not have the same local resources, but don't worry.**

**There are online resources** like *www.azurestandard.com* and *www.thrivemarket.com*, both of which I have used for years. You can also use the links in this article to look for farmers and other alternative food, meat, and water resources closer to you: *www.sharonharmon.com/blog/alternative-food-sources*.

And, don't forget, you can find more specific items and brands in my free resource, *Natural Pantry Checklist*. Download it from my website at *www.sharonharmon.com/freebies*.

Now that you have learned many tips about shopping free of gluten, dairy, and GMOs, let's move on to baking. When you know how to convert your favorite recipes to gluten-free options, it can be a game changer and less overwhelming to move forward, especially with children.

## Chapter 5 Summary

∞ Not all gluten-free (and dairy-free) products are created equal. Many contain oats, which are not inherently gluten-free. Plus there is a wide spectrum of "health food" products, so learn to be selective.

∞ Consider how the food is packaged as toxic packaging can get into the foods they contain, especially when purchasing oils and greasy products.

∞ Genetically modified (or GMO) ingredients are commonly found in packaged and processed foods, so read the ingredients carefully. GMO crops, like corn and soy, can be used as grains as well as oils, sugars, binders, additives, and even fortified vitamins.

∞ To truly heal your digestive system, you need to be conscious of all your food decisions including prewashed produce, condiment selection, drink options, fortified products, and meat/cheese substitutes. (See Chapter 5 for details.)

∞ Optimally, the foods you eat should be as close to their naturally grown state as possible. Any processed foods, like crackers or milk alternatives, should have minimal ingredients and no additives.

∞ Any animal products, like eggs, meat, and fish (including dairy), should be from trusted sources where animals are grass-fed, pastured, wild-caught (no farmed fish), and not given pharmaceuticals. If feed is given to an animal, it should be gluten-free and GMO-free.

∞ Bread and other baked goods can be especially difficult to find gluten-free, dairy-free, and GMO-free but there are a few options. When necessary, compare available products and find the best option (concentrating on gluten-free and corn-free) with the fewest ingredients, and eat in moderation.

# CHAPTER 6

# Baking Gluten-free (and Dairy-free)

Growing up, I was the baker in the family. Being the only daughter in a family of seven, I did not have much competition, so it was often me who made the desserts and birthday cakes.

Back then, to make a recipe "healthier" meant using whole-wheat flour instead of white flour and replacing sugar with honey. I loved baking as well as sharing and eating the results!

As an adult when my family started eating gluten-free, I took my love of baking and used it to experiment. I converted my favorite recipes into healthy gluten-free and dairy-free options. That means GMO-free too.

The biggest challenge was finding the right combination of gluten-free flours. Eventually, I figured out a few secrets that took my creations to a new level, as I will explain in this chapter.

**Baking gluten-free can be challenging at first, but it is very doable**. And, making food at home is definitely preferable if you are going to eat gluten-free the right way. You control every ingredient.

Once you realize you can easily convert your current favorite recipes into gluten-free favorites, changing out culprit ingredients for good, healthy ones, everyone in the family will be on board.

I once took a complicated Kraft™ recipe for German chocolate cake that my mother-in-law made annually for my husband's birthday and made it gluten-free and dairy-free. Even the skeptics in the family admitted it tasted good. I know it can be done.

The good news is that there are many more gluten-free recipes available online than when I first got started. However, you need to be discerning as each person's definition of "gluten-free" is different. Some recipes use oats, for example.

You also need to consider other culprit foods and GMOs as discussed in this book. So, when using online recipes, you may still need to substitute suspect ingredients with the ones explained in this chapter.

This is why I created my own healthy cookbook that is gluten-free, dairy-free, and GMO-free, which you can find on my website at *www.sharonharmon.com/books*. It corresponds to all the information I give you in this book. (You can find the German chocolate cake recipe in there too.) It is a helpful healing tool. It includes baked goods as well as hot meals, soups, salads/dressings, beverages, snacks, and so much more.

## Basic Baking Concepts

Initially, when we went gluten-free and dairy-free, my baking wonders were not so wonderful. Replacing dairy ingredients with coconut versions was not difficult, especially with all the new options that have become available the last several years. However, replacing the flour was a little more challenging, especially when using natural sweeteners.

I have experimented with all sorts of flours. Initially, I strictly used rice flour (which is inherently gluten-free) and replaced all the required flour in a recipe with rice flour. However, the resulting treat was always too crumbly. I also tried other gluten-free flours like garbanzo bean flour and quinoa flakes without much difference.

A common trend in gluten-free baking is to add xanthan gum, which acts very much like the gluten in wheat and binds the ingredients together, but I am **not a big fan of xanthan gum**, as I have mentioned before.

First of all, it is most often derived from corn or soy, both genetically modified (GM) crops (corn with the Bt toxin). Xanthan gum is also made by a bacterial fermentation process. I have found it to be a common stomach irritant. It should also not be given to babies whose digestive systems are not fully developed. Why chance it?

Nut flours were not as difficult to bake with but still resulted in a crumblier version of the original. Over time, I also came to realize that we were eating way too many nuts. In my family, we ate soaked and dehydrated nuts daily. If I baked with them as well, that was too much. (See more about nuts and oxalates in Chapter 4.)

I also started to question how healthy ground nuts were after being cooked in the oven since heat can make the oil in the nuts rancid.

For a while, we went grain-free, so I tried baking with coconut flour. Although this is a good option if eating grain-free, coconut flour is nothing like grain-based flours. It soaks up so much liquid that you have to rethink the whole recipe, so it is best to go with a proven coconut flour recipe rather than directly substituting, as I explain below.

## Experimenting and Discoveries

Eventually, I had two big epiphanies: (1) I eventually created a good, simple flour combination and (2) I determined I needed to modify the oven temperature. I discuss these and a few other tips below.

***Gluten-free Flour*** – I have found that if I combine **rice flour with tapioca flour**, the tapioca helps hold together the baked goods better. Whenever a recipe calls for flour, replace that quantity proportionally with three-quarters rice flour and one-quarter tapioca flour (or another binder as explained below).

I originally tried this combination in multiple recipes during the Christmas holidays and in several birthday cakes, and it worked great every time. My results were moist and not crumbly.

If you want to vary your flours, as I recommend when eating gluten-free, other common "gluten-free" flours include **amaranth, buckwheat, millet, quinoa, and sorghum**. Note, however, that some of these have a distinctive taste that not everyone may appreciate. Use organic whenever possible.

Notice that I did not include corn or soy in this list. Although both are inherently gluten-free, both are common GMO crops, especially in the United States. (Corn crops are easily cross-pollinated, so even organic options may be tainted. See Chapter 3 for more information.)

I also did not include oats on this list because it too has gluten. In reality, all grains have different types of gluten (as explained in Chapter 1), but I have found that oat gluten is too close to wheat gluten, so it is usually best to avoid it if you are gluten-free, especially in the beginning stages.

If you do use oats (or groats), or decide to add them back into your diet later on, be sure to purchase a brand that is guaranteed gluten-free since they are often processed in facilities that process wheat. It should also be organic since standard oats are typically sprayed with the pesticide glyphosate right before harvesting.

**Grain-free Flours** – There are grain-free flour options as well. The most common include **almond flour, cassava flour, chickpea (garbanzo bean) flour, and coconut flour**. More options are becoming available as well, like **tiger nut flour and green banana flour**. (Tiger nut flour is actually from a small root vegetable.)

If you use almond or other nut flour, it is typically a one-to-one substitute for regular flour. However, as I explained in Chapter 4, it is best to limit the amount of nut flours in your gluten-free diet.

Cassava and chickpea (or garbanzo bean) flour also typically have a one-to-one ratio. However, some of these flours have a more distinctive taste than others, so you may need to experiment. Use them in different combinations or use some of the binders mentioned below, such as tapioca and arrowroot (which are also grain-free), to minimize the taste.

Coconut flour tends to be a little trickier to use because it really absorbs the liquid in a recipe. It can be difficult to get the liquid proportions correct. The typical rule is that 1/4 cup of coconut flour equals a full cup of all-purpose flour. Any more than that and your creations will be too dry, unless you include additional liquid and/or eggs. You should also let your batter set for 15 or 20 minutes before baking so the coconut absorbs the liquid before you put it into the oven.

**Binders** – In addition to the tapioca flour mentioned above, **arrowroot flour, potato starch/flour, and guar gum** (made from a seed) are also considered gluten-free and can be used as a binder or thickener. Some use **psyllium hulls** as well. A binder helps hold the ingredients together better, since gluten-free baked goods tend to be crumblier.

I avoid **xanthan gum** for the reasons I explained above. Guar gum may also be questionable for people with sensitive digestive systems. If you want to avoid the binders, making mini-muffins or mini-cupcakes helps to eliminate crumbling issues. It is a great alternative for treats. (Using additional eggs in a recipe can also act as a binder, but you would need to adjust the liquids in the recipe.)

**Sweeteners** – I used to bake with honey, but I could tell that I personally needed to change to a different sweetener. For some reason when baked, the honey gave me too much of a sugar "rush." Sometimes I use maple syrup.

My favorite sweetener is coconut sugar or coconut palm sugar. Both are known to have a lower glycemic index than cane sugar. Other favorites include rapadura sugar or date sugar. (Avoid monk fruit with erythritol, or other artificial sugars as discussed in Chapter 5. Pure monk fruit is available but highly sweet so you need very little of it in a recipe.)

The more natural sugars are typically darker, so if you are not careful, they tend to make baked goods darker, burn easier, and drier to the taste. My fix for this is to bake the recipe at a lower temperature than suggested, typically 25 degrees lower. If the recipe calls for 350F degrees, for example, I use 325F degrees and cook for about the same amount of time.

Depending on the recipe, you may need a few minutes longer than what is suggested, so keep a good watch at the end to make sure it does not get too dark.

**Dairy** – If a recipe calls for milk-type products, there are plenty of coconut product options. I like it best as it is creamier than other dairy substitutes and has a consistency closest to milk. And, unlike coconut flour, the coconut taste goes away in most recipes.

I avoid soy milks because of the GMOs and the additives. I also limit the use of oat and nut milks for the same reasons I mentioned above. Some people are okay eating butter, but if you need a butter substitute you can use ghee or coconut oil. See below for additional dairy substitutes.

## My Favorite Substitutes

When I bake gluten-free, dairy-free, and GMO-free, I tend to make it as simple as possible. I also use organic ingredients whenever I can. If you are in the beginning stages of eating gluten-free, the key is to **start replacing the items in your pantry one item at a time**. Begin with the items you use most often.

Below is a list of what I typically use in baking recipes. (For brand names, download my free resource, *Natural Pantry Checklist*, found on my website at *www.sharonharmon.com/freebies*.)

**Sugar** = coconut sugar or rapadura sugar
(Date sugar is another good one because it is full of minerals, but it is harder to find. I still use honey or maple syrup once in a while, but then you have to modify the liquids and/or dry ingredients to accommodate the liquid sweetener. If you use cane sugar, be sure

it is organic because most cane crops are sprayed with the herbicide glyphosate right before harvesting.)

**Flour** = Combination of rice flour and tapioca flour in 3:1 ratio (see previous section)
(I try to use sprouted rice flour whenever I can because that is easier to digest than regular rice flour. For a heartier flavor, I sometimes use sprouted garbanzo bean flour, instead of tapioca, especially when making pancakes. I alternate between using brown rice and white rice flour to create more variety.)

**Milk** = Coconut milk
(Look for brands that do not line their cans with plastic and ones with limited ingredients. There are options without guar gum as a thickener, but it may not be creamy enough for some recipes.)

**Buttermilk** = Coconut milk with lemon juice added
(Use 1 to 2 teaspoons of fresh-squeezed lemon juice with every cup of coconut milk.)

**Evaporated Milk** = Condensed coconut milk
(Yes, this is actually an available product.)

**Heavy Cream** = Coconut Cream
(Another great find. It can even be blended to make whipped cream.)

**Butter** = Ghee (clarified butter)
(You can also use oil or coconut shortening instead of butter, see below. Applesauce in a 1:1 ratio is another option if you want to avoid the fat. Stay away from margarine since most are made with hydrogenated oils and/or GM soy.)

**Oil** = Coconut oil or avocado oil
(Never use conventional vegetable oils or seed oils. Don't bake

with olive oil since it has a low-temperature smoke point. Find out more about healthy oils, the best ways to use them, and which ones to avoid at *www.sharonharmon.com/blog/good-fats-and-oils.*)

**Shortening** = Coconut-based shortening
(Stay away from conventional brands, which are typically made with hydrogenated oils.)

If you happen to be **sensitive to eggs**, there are several egg substitutes available. Be selective of the ones you purchase in the store as some have suspect ingredients. You can easily make your own, see *www.sharonharmon.com/blog/egg-substitutes.*

For more ideas on healthy gluten-free, dairy-free, and GMO-free baking products and brands, download my free resource, *Natural Pantry Checklist,* found at *www.sharonharmon.com/freebies.*

And be sure to check out my companion cookbook that is gluten-free, dairy-free, and GMO-free and follows all the concepts in this book. Find it on my website at *www.sharonharmon.com/books.* It includes a collection of simple recipes for everyday life.

Eating healthy does not need to be boring. However, I would still caution you not to go overboard when it comes to baking. Even healthy homemade treats and desserts should be limited, only eaten after getting in your daily fruits, vegetables, proteins, fats, and other nutritious foods.

# Chapter 6 Summary

∞ Baking gluten-free (and dairy-free) can be challenging at first, but once you learn the basics, you can convert your existing favorite recipes, which is especially helpful when children are involved.

∞ To get the best results when baking, it is best to use a combination of gluten-free flour. This allows for better binding, less crumbling, and optimal flavor. (See suggestions in Chapter 6.)

∞ Using a lower-than-normal oven temperature when baking can also be helpful.

∞ Binders are key to gluten-free baking since you are missing the wheat gluten that makes typical baked goods fluffier and chewier. Gluten-free examples include arrowroot flour, potato starch, and psyllium hulls.

∞ Binders like xanthan gum, and even guar gum for some, can be a stomach irritant. Plus xanthan gum is often made from GMO corn so it is optimal not to use it, especially if you are in the early stages of healing.

∞ When you are healing your gut, sweeteners should also be kept to a minimum. More natural options include coconut sugar, date sugar, maple syrup, and rapadura sugar.

∞ Dairy-free substitutes are easy with all the coconut-milk-based products available. Most people can tolerate ghee if they need to remove butter from their diet.

∞ Baking at home can be a great way to include quality gluten-free options that are difficult to find in a store, but don't go overboard. Even healthy baked goods are not good if eaten in abundance.

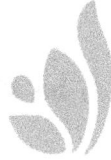

# Where to Go from Here

If you already started your gluten-free, dairy-free, and GMO-free journey, congratulations! Use this book to tweak your daily eating habits and discover what you may need to change to get the results you want.

If all of this is brand new, and it feels a bit overwhelming, not to worry. Go through one chapter of this book at a time, and take baby steps. You did not start eating a certain way all at once. **Give yourself permission to take it one step at a time.** Find your worst culprit foods and start there.

In fact, it **may be best to start with going GMO-free**, since these genetically modified and high pesticide and herbicide foods are part of the reason our digestive systems are so compromised in the first place. By eliminating these foods first, your gut has a better chance of healing as you eliminate the gluten and/or dairy. As I have explained throughout the book, healing your digestive system is a big part of the solution.

After reviewing the lifestyle factors in Chapter 2, you may realize that **some of your daily habits affect your digestive system**. For example, you may be texting regularly with your cell phone near your stomach or using a laptop against your body. You may need to stop drinking tap water or resolve a stressful situation. See which lifestyle habits you need to modify as you also shift your eating habits.

**So, how long do you need to be gluten-free, dairy-free, and GMO-free?**

Well, the answer is **different for everyone**. It will depend on the state of your health when you start eliminating foods, how strict you are during the process, how many other lifestyle factors you address, and how proactive you are with gut healing.

I believe everyone should be GMO-free, or as much as possible, for a lifetime, for the many reasons I explain in this book. Gluten (and dairy), on the other hand, will depend. Many people do feel better if they permanently stay away from gluten. You may find that your body is okay with certain grains or foods after taking a break from them and improving your overall food and lifestyle choices.

In my family, for example, I continue to shop and cook free of gluten, dairy, and GMOs at home. (We do use quality butter regularly.) Other family members will eat differently when eating elsewhere, like at a restaurant or a friend's house. However, I remain GMO-free, gluten-free, and mostly dairy-free. I may have raw cheese once in a while, especially when I can find a good source, but that is it.

I feel better eating this way and have learned how to participate in life to the fullest while eating with family and friends, going out to eat, traveling with family or for work, etc. It may take some planning, but it is now second nature to me. I have a complicated health history, including taking antibiotics for 6 years as a child, and did not start eating this way until my 40s. It makes sense for my lifestyle and body.

As my son got older, started driving, and becoming more independent, he decided to broaden his food choices. He eats out regularly with his friends, eating gluten and dairy. We worked hard on building his gut and eliminating toxins (see Chapter 2) during the years he was not consuming gluten, dairy, and GMOs. I also taught him the many concepts in this book. He knows how to be selective when necessary. He can recognize his unique physical and emotional symptoms, and knows when he needs to get temporarily stricter with his food choices.

There are many other scenarios, each specific to the person. I have clients, for example, who only need to be gluten-free and dairy-free for 3, 6, or 18 months as they heal their gut lining and other specific symptoms by removing toxins, microbes, and stress while working on their digestive system. This often works for younger children as well.

Other people may be able to introduce raw dairy but feel better remaining gluten-free. Or, maybe add homemade yogurt and/or kefir, which can be very healing for the digestive system. They continue to remain GMO-free as much as possible, especially avoiding processed foods containing corn and soy, since these are big culprit foods for many people.

Depending on your or your child's particular health situation, it **may be best to work with a knowledgeable alternative practitioner**, one who has experience with food elimination and/or gut healing. Eliminating food can be very healing in and of itself, but more often, additional steps need to be taken to heal the gut. This allows you to reintroduce certain foods sooner and avoid potential nutritional deficiencies.

Supplements can be helpful when healing the gut. However, which supplements to take will depend on the person. Each situation is different because each of us is unique. You have your unique health history, family or generational weaknesses, environmental triggers, traumas, etc.

With the right practitioner, you can also attend to the other lifestyle factors discussed in Chapter 2. Are there toxins you need to eliminate from your daily life and/or from your body? Is there a low-grade infection going on that you are not aware of? Are there current stressors or older traumas that need to be resolved? The more you consider and address, the healthier you become.

As you heal and start feeling better, my hope is that you get to a point where you know intuitively what to do. Or, you experiment by adding in foods a little at a time, after you have been strict, whether it is for the 2-week elimination period or the full 3, 6 to 18 months, and see how you feel. As you slowly reintroduce foods, pay attention to your body's reaction. Keep a journal. Your body will tell you what it can tolerate when you pay attention.

**The good news is that the body can heal. It was designed that way! We just need to give it the right tools**.

Learn more about your body and more natural lifestyle habits on my website *www.sharonharmon.com*. There are many free resources available.

# Resources

*Gluten-free the Right Way!* is a great primer explaining the why and how of going gluten-free. If you want to research gluten further and learn more about the science or how to get tested, below are some of my favorite resources.

As you move forward in your journey, remember what you learned in this book. You will find that there are a variety of "gluten" experts and some will be more well-versed than others.

With *Gluten-free the Right Way!*, you will be ready to think outside the box and ask questions that are specific to you and your situation.

## Gluten-free Resources

### *Books for Further Research*

*You Can Fix Your Brain*, Dr. Tom O'Brien
*No Grain, No Pain*, Dr. Peter Osborne
*Grain Brain*, Dr. David Perlmutter

### *Testing Options*

*www.cyrex.com*
*www.thedr.com* (includes "Certified Gluten-free Practitioner" listing)
*www.glutenfreesociety.org* (includes Gluten Sensitivity Quiz)

### *Other Gluten-free Resources*

*www.beyondceliac.org*
*www.gfco.org* (certification and labeling)

# GMO-free Resources

*www.responsibletechnology.org* (most current GM information)
*www.nongmoproject.org* (certification and labeling)
*www.whatsonmyfood.org* (more pesticide-related)
*www.livecornfree.com* (lists corn-containing foods)

# Other Suggested Books

*The Elimination Diet*, Alissa Segersten and Tom Malterre
*Toxic Superfoods*, Sally Norton (more about oxalates)
*The Biology of Belief*, Dr. Bruce Lipton

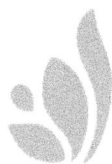

# About the Author

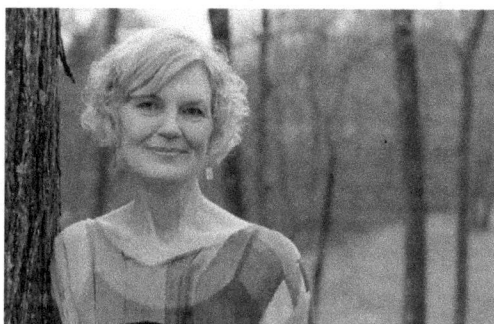

Sharon K. Harmon, PhD received her master's and doctorate in Holistic Health after a winding health journey of her own. Learning early on that traditional medical interventions did not work for her and later discovering she is what is known as a "highly sensitive person," Sharon learned to think outside the box when it came to health. Her sensitivities caused her body to react to her food and the environment more quickly than others. Over the years this included building toxins, heavy metals, Lyme, electromagnetic frequencies (EMFs), mold. . . and gluten.

Sharon is on a mission to help families and other highly sensitive people find their path to good health. She believes improving the foods we eat is an important step in the process.

# Invitation

For more valuable health-related resources, tips, and tools, including online classes, to help you on your health journey, please join me at *www.sharonharmon.com*. I invite you to learn more about your body and the environment around you, so that you can take your health to the next level.

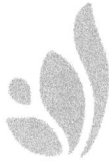

# Please Leave a Review

Thank you for reading this book. I hope you enjoyed it and are well on your way to better health.

Now, I would like to ask you a small favor. Would you kindly take a moment to leave a review on Amazon? Here is a short link to make it easier for you: *https://a.co/d/flfyUDH*

It would mean a great deal to me, and I am grateful for the time you take to write it!

Blessings, Sharon

www.ingramcontent.com/pod-product-compliance
Lightning Source LLC
Chambersburg PA
CBHW052139270326
41930CB00012B/2948